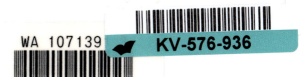
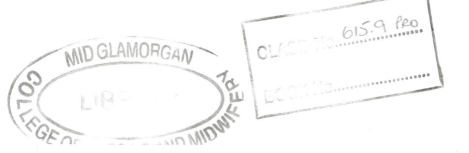
**This book is to be returned on or before
the last date stamped below.**

Acute Poisoning

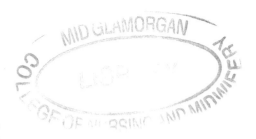

Acute Poisoning

Diagnosis and management

Second edition

A. T. Proudfoot
Director, Scottish Poisons Information Bureau

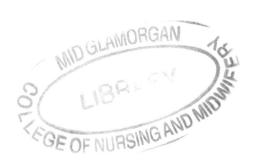

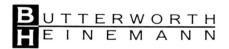

BUTTERWORTH
HEINEMANN

615.9 PRO

Butterworth-Heinemann Ltd
Linacre House, Jordan Hill, Oxford OX2 8DP

 A member of the Reed Elsevier group

OXFORD LONDON BOSTON
MUNICH NEW DELHI SINGAPORE SYDNEY
TOKYO TORONTO WELLINGTON

First published by Blackwell Scientific Publications 1982
Second edition published by Butterworth-Heinemann Ltd 1993

British Library Cataloguing in Publication Data
Proudfoot, A. T.
 Acute Poisoning: Diagnosis and
 Management. – 2Rev. ed
 I. Title
 615.9

ISBN 0 7506 1445 5

Composition by Genesis Typesetting, Laser Quay, Rochester, Kent
Printed and bound in Great Britain by Biddles Ltd, Guildford and King's Lynn

12/11/93

Contents

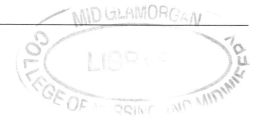

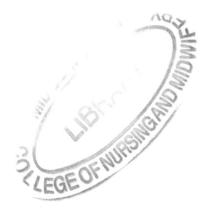

Preface

Acute poisoning remains one of the most common medical emergencies and responsibility for its immediate management continues to fall mainly on junior doctors in emergency departments and medical units. It is at them that this book is principally directed but hopefully senior medical students and postgraduates will also find it useful.

Clinical toxicology has advanced considerably in the ten years since this book first appeared. Amongst other things, the pattern of poisoning has changed, the value of some traditional treatments has been challenged and found seriously wanting, new therapies have arrived and, in general, the discipline is now subject to much more critical and scientific appraisal. I doubt if every doctor is aware of these improvements and I continue to hope that this book will stimulate them to a more thoughtful approach to the diagnosis and management of poisoned patients.

The book is essentially a practical guide and is therefore fairly dogmatic. Although the format remains unchanged, the contents have been radically revised, obsolete material deleted and much that is new added. As before, the references quoted are as up to date as possible and even if they are not necessarily the most useful, they will guide readers to the earlier literature.

My special thanks go to Mrs Alison Good, without whose support in general and expertise in word processing and bibliographic searching in particular, I would have been driven to despair. I also thank Miss Jacqueline West for her assiduousness in tracking down many of the references quoted.

A.T. Proudfoot

Chapter 1

Acute poisoning – definition and classification

Definition

'Poisoning' is an emotive term which demands definition if it is not to be applied indiscriminately. The *Oxford English Dictionary* (2nd edition, 1989) states that a poison is 'any substance which when introduced into, or absorbed by, a living organism destroys life or injures health irrespective of mechanical means or direct thermal changes'. Acceptance of this definition requires one to accept that:

1 *Exposures which do not cause unwelcome and adverse consequences whether experienced by the individual or identified in him or her by others, are not 'poisonings'.* Such incidents are now more accurately termed 'non-toxic exposures'.
2 *Side-effects of therapeutic doses of drugs are also manifestations of 'poisoning'.* While accepting this definition, one must acknowledge that the increase in information on the side-effects of therapeutic agents has been so great that this aspect of poisoning has become an independent discipline encompassed under the heading of adverse reactions and is the province of clinical pharmacology. Clinical (human) toxicology deals with the everyday incidents involving exposure to excessive doses of drugs or to substances never intended to be ingested, inhaled, or to be applied to the skin or eyes which are perhaps more commonly perceived as 'poisonings'.
3 *Chemically inert substances are 'poisons' if their introduction into the body obstructs internal passages and causes symptoms and/or signs.*

Classification

Poisoning episodes may be classified into four types, of which only two are common. Although most poisoning episodes can be readily allocated to one of these categories, occasionally classification may be difficult.

This is particularly the case when trying to decide whether mild intoxication in elderly patients has been the result of confusion and therapeutic misadventure or deliberate self-poisoning. Similarly overdosage in drug addicts is often regarded as accidental but could equally be classified as self-poisoning. The latter view is recommended.

Accidental

Accidental poisoning may be encountered at any age but the causes differ.

Neonatal poisoning

Neonates may be born poisoned as a result of therapeutic doses of drugs or self-poisoning (defined below) in the late stages of labour. Congenital poisoning with salicylates, benzodiazepines and opioid analgesics is well documented. However, neonates are at particular risk because of their environments (e.g. incubators and intensive care units) and therapeutic errors on the part of their carers. Thus some have received ergometrine intended for their mothers and others have been given excessive amounts of drugs as a result of miscalculation of doses. Therapeutic misadventure is the term commonly applied to such incidents.

Children

Accidental poisoning is most frequently encountered in children between the ages of 1 and 5 years and is the usual cause of poisoning in this age group. It is the consequence of newly acquired independent mobility, innate curiosity and a predilection for exploring the environment with the mouth as well as the eyes and fingers. It is commonly held that adults facilitate this form of poisoning by leaving household cleaning agents, toiletries and drugs within easy reach in cupboards, beneath kitchen sinks, on bedside tables and in unlocked bathroom cabinets. However, accidental poisoning in childhood is not simply a matter of overactivity and ready accessibility of poisons. Homes in which a child poisoning occurs are no more dangerous in terms of availability of potential poisons but are much more likely to have been disturbed by a recent house removal, pregnancy, physical or mental illness in one of the parents or by one parent being away from home. These events may predispose to poisoning episodes by reducing supervision of the children.

Older children and adults

Accidental poisoning may occur in older children and adults particularly as a result of mishaps at school or work, e.g. inhalation of gases such as chlorine or fumes from organic solvents, ingestion of chemical reagents while pipetting, or drinking some toxic fluid which has been decanted into a soft-drink or beer bottle.

Accidental poisoning with drugs may also occur in confused elderly patients prescribed large numbers of medicines. They may forget the dose and frequency with which each should be taken and make mistakes. While the underlying problem may be dementia, confusion and forgetfulness are frequently aggravated or precipitated by inappropriate psychotropic medication.

'Body packing' is also a potential cause of accidental poisoning in adults. This term refers to the practice of smuggling drugs by concealing them in body cavities. The drugs are commonly packaged in contraceptive sheaths or in cellophane or metallic foil wrappings and swallowed or inserted into the rectum or vagina. The practitioners of body packing are sometimes referred to as 'mules' and their subdivision into 'swallowers' and 'stuffers' is self-explanatory. Clearly, they are at risk of poisoning if the contents of packages leak.

Deliberate self-poisoning

Deliberate self-poisoning is the commonest form of poisoning in adults and accounts for at least 95% of all poisoning admissions to hospital. It is sometimes referred to as attempted suicide, parasuicide or pseudocide and is more common in women. Such patients intentionally take poisons or overdoses of drugs, often impulsively, after a disagreement with a key person in their lives. At the moment of crisis little or no thought is given to the risk and the possible outcome is of no immediate concern. Most patients, however, have no wish to die. They soon regret their actions and willingly seek medical help. A minority of adults who poison themselves are intent on dying and carefully plan the event, ascertaining as far as possible the toxicity and likely fatal dose of a drug, accumulating a sufficient quantity and taking it under circumstances which make intervention by others improbable. These patients are usually profoundly depressed or psychotic. Another small group of adults deliberately takes poisons to teach others a lesson or to manipulate them into an attitude or course of action that they would otherwise reject.

The peak age incidence for self-poisoning is between 20 and 35 years, but it is not uncommon before the age of 15 years. Self-poisoning should be suspected in any episode occurring over the age of 8 years.

Non-accidental poisoning

Non-accidental poisoning, a variety of Münchausen syndrome by proxy, is the term given to the deliberate administration of a poison to a child by one of its parents and may be regarded as an extension of the battered child syndrome. It may be more common than is generally appreciated. The causes are not clear, but there is usually disharmony between the parents and the child's illness may be used by one parent to distress the other or to help reduce marital tension by making the child the focus of attention.

Homicidal poisoning

Acute poisoning as a method of homicide is very uncommon. Sporadic cases occur but in most the poisoning is subacute or chronic as with antimony, arsenic and thallium.

Points of emphasis

- Incidents involving exposure to potential poisons but which are not followed by symptoms or signs should be termed non-toxic exposures and not poisonings.
- Accidental poisoning is most frequent between the ages of 1 and 5 years.
- Self-poisoning should be considered in any episode over the age of 8 years but the peak incidence is between 20 and 35 years.
- Most adults who poison themselves act impulsively and have no wish to die.
- Homicidal poisoning is rare but non-accidental poisoning in children may be more common than is generally appreciated.

Chapter 2

Diagnosis of poisoning

In the great majority of cases, a diagnosis of acute poisoning is reached on the history given by the patient, by a witness to the episode or on circumstantial evidence. The findings on physical examination may help corroborate the nature of the suspected poison but, in isolation, are seldom sufficiently characteristic to make an unassailable diagnosis of poisoning. The diagnosis can, of course, be made in the absence of any history, circumstantial evidence or typical physical signs by finding high plasma concentrations of drugs, though comprehensive laboratory screening services are available in only a few centres.

History

Adults

About 90% of adults who take poisons are conscious on arrival at hospital, and it is not usually difficult to elicit a history of self-poisoning.

Nature of the poison

Patients' statements about the nature of the poisons ingested should be accepted with caution since the drugs found on analysis of blood or urine often correlate poorly with those alleged to have been taken. As a result, some clinicians believe that patients are at best completely unreliable or at worst deliberately misleading. Undoubtedly some do lie about the nature of the drug or poison taken, but the majority are probably as truthful as their knowledge permits. Many patients do not know what they have taken, because they took the first tablets that came to hand and in about 15% of cases these have been prescribed for some other person. Incredibly, others blithely take unnamed drugs bought or offered free in public houses in the expectation they will make them 'feel good'. Intoxication with alcohol at the time of self-poisoning is a common reason for ignorance of the poison taken. To some extent the nature of the drug may be corroborated by descriptions of the tablets or capsules, identification of remaining pills or from labels on containers.

While an element of scepticism about patients' statements is clinically healthy there is often no choice but to accept them since it would be impracticable, expensive and unnecessary to obtain laboratory confirmation in every case.

Quantity of the poison
Statements about the quantity of poison taken are even more open to question. A minority of individuals deliberately exaggerate or understate the quantity they have taken according to whether they wish to attract attention or play down the episode. Most, however, are uncertain about quantities simply because they do not count the number of tablets but take them by the handful, not knowing how many were in the bottle in the first place. Again uncertainty about quantity is often due to the influence of alcohol.

Unconscious patients
When adults are found unconscious and a history is not available, a diagnosis of poisoning involves the exclusion of other causes of coma (p. 17) and consideration of circumstantial evidence. The possibility of poisoning must never be dismissed because of the protestations of relatives that the patient would never take an overdose or that no drugs were available. Close relatives are often the last to recognize emotional distress in other members of the household. It must be remembered that drug overdosage is one of the commonest causes of coma in young and middle-aged adults.

Drug overdosage is virtually certain if individuals are found unconscious with empty tablet bottles or a few tablets scattered nearby. When gas is used, the patient may have tried to seal gaps around doors and windows. Suicide notes often make their actions and intentions clear. On other occasions patients may go to unusual places or to remote countryside to take overdoses and may deliberately divest themselves of objects that might identify them should they be discovered. The absence of such identifying articles should raise the suspicion of poisoning.

Reference
Ray JE, Reilly DK, Day RO. Drugs involved in self-poisoning: verification by toxicological analysis. *Med J Aust* 1986; **144**: 455–457.

Children

Accidental poisoning in children is usually a matter of conjecture. A toddler may be found with an open container and/or with hands, face, clothing and surrounding floor soiled with some household product or disintegrated tablets. Under these circumstances it is reasonable to assume that some may have been ingested. In other cases an older child may report that a poison has been taken. In the absence of a witness to the act of poisoning the diagnosis may be suspected from abnormal behaviour, convulsions, ataxia or gastrointestinal disturbances.

Reference

Fazen LE, Lovejoy FH, Crone RK. Acute poisoning in a children's hospital: a 2-year experience. *Pediatrics* 1986; **77**: 144–151.

Deliberate poisoning of others

Homicidal poisoning and non-accidental poisoning may be extremely difficult to recognize and require a high index of suspicion. Adults may express the fear that they are being poisoned but young children cannot. In the latter inexplicable features, particularly convulsions, drowsiness and staggering occurring in an episodic manner, should arouse suspicion. Complete recovery usually occurs after removal from the home environment but symptoms may recur after discharge or even while in hospital. In the latter case they can be related to a parental visit. Careful questioning may reveal suspicious deaths or illness in siblings, availability of drugs to parents and psychological stresses in the family. A history of self-poisoning or drug misuse in the parents is not unusual.

References

Alexander R, Smith W, Stevenson R. Serial Munchausen syndrome by proxy. *Pediatrics* 1990; **86**: 581–585.
Hickson GB, Altemeier WA, Martin ED *et al.* Parental administration of chemical agents: a cause of apparent life-threatening events. *Pediatrics* 1989; **83**: 772–776.

Symptoms and signs

Most poisoned adults are able to tell what has been taken and symptoms are of relatively little diagnostic value. However, their presence or absence may give some indication of the severity of poisoning. Many poisons affect multiple body systems and symptoms are frequently numerous and non-specific. Similarly, physical signs appear in clusters rather than singly and are of particular importance in establishing a diagnosis in unconscious patients.

Reference

Olson KR, Pentel PR, Kelley MT. Physical assessment and differential diagnosis of the poisoned patient. *Med Toxicol* 1987; **2**: 52–81.

Alimentary features

Pain and ulceration of the oral cavity

Pain and ulceration of the mouth, throat and tongue follow the ingestion of strong alkalis or acids which are the common constituents of drain and pipe cleaners and descalers. Among the most common are solutions of paraquat, phenols and sodium hydroxide. Domestic bleaches are also alkaline but are not sufficiently strong to produce much mucosal damage or mouth pain. Strong acids produce similar symptoms, but though phenols and cresols (as in Lysol) cause buccal burns they are generally painless because of destruction of pain fibres. The burns may not be obvious for 24–36 hours.

Salivation

Increased salivation is occasionally seen in patients who have ingested corrosive agents or large quantities of chlormethiazole, phencyclidine, cholinesterase inhibitors (organophosphate and carbamate insecticides) and inorganic iodides and bromides. The last-named may also cause enlargement of the salivary glands.

Dry mouth

Dryness of the tongue and mouth is often due to anticholinergic compounds but must be interpreted with caution in the presence of mouth-breathing and hyperventilation.

Dysphagia

Pain or difficulty in swallowing may simply be due to dryness of the mouth and throat as above but can also complicate ingestion of foreign bodies and corrosive agents. Clinitest tablets may become adherent to the buccal and oesophageal mucosa and cause burns by virtue of their sodium hydroxide content. Denture cleaning tablets cause similar problems because of their size and content of sodium perborate, trisodium phosphate and sodium carbonate.

Nausea and vomiting

Nausea and vomiting are probably the most common non-specific alimentary symptoms of poisoning. They may be due to direct irritation of the gastric mucosa or to a central effect after absorption of some drugs including opioid analgesics, theophylline derivatives and digoxin. In such cases nausea and vomiting usually come on within a few hours.

If the onset is delayed for 24–36 hours other causes such as hepatic necrosis, pancreatitis or renal failure may be responsible.

Abdominal pain and diarrhoea
Generalized abdominal pain and diarrhoea starting shortly after ingestion are usually due to corrosives or drugs which irritate the gastrointestinal tract, e.g. strong alkalis and acids, mercuric chloride, iron salts, laxatives or colchicine. Pain which is delayed in onset is often more localized, right subcostal discomfort usually being due to hepatic damage and bilateral loin or renal angle pain to renal tubular necrosis.

Loss of bowel sounds
Reduction of bowel sounds often occurs in patients who are deeply unconscious but abdominal distension and ileus are rare. Opioid analgesics and anticholinergic compounds are particularly likely to abolish bowel sounds but activity returns rapidly as consciousness is regained.

Jaundice
Hepatocellular jaundice due to poisons takes 2–3 days to develop and is, therefore, of little diagnostic value since most patients are admitted within 24 hours of the poisoning. Paracetamol is by far the most commonly encountered hepatotoxin. Carbon tetrachloride, other halogenated hydrocarbons, phenylbutazone and the death-cap mushroom, *Amanita phalloides*, should also be considered. Less commonly, jaundice may be due to haemolysis by chlorate, nomifensine or arsine.

Reference

Mueller PD, Benowitz NL. Toxicologic causes of acute abdominal disorders. *Emerg Med Clin North Am* 1989; 7: 667–682.

Cerebral and neuromuscular features

Staggering and dizziness
Overdoses of central nervous system (CNS) depressants cause staggering, dizziness, stiffness and weakness. These symptoms are the result of neuromuscular incoordination which can be confirmed by demonstrating nystagmus or carrying out the finger–nose test.

Coma
Coma is one of the most common signs of poisoning and is usually due to direct CNS depression by hypnotics, antidepressants, other anticholinergic drugs, anticonvulsants, tranquillizers, opioid analgesics,

alcohols and glycols. It is an uncommon feature of severe salicylate poisoning and does not occur with paracetamol intoxication unless another drug such as dextropropoxyphene (as in co-proxamol) has been taken simultaneously or hepatic encephalopathy has developed. Many hydrocarbons are volatile and lipid-soluble and may cause coma when ingested (e.g. trichloroethane, trichloroethylene and other dry-cleaning and degreasing agents) or inhaled (as with most substances sniffed by those who abuse volatile substances). Coma may also be caused indirectly by hypoglycaemia following administration of insulin and sulphonylureas.

Muscle tone and reflex changes
Hypotonia and hyporeflexia are usual with overdosage of benzodiazepines, barbiturates, most other hypnotics and phenothiazines. Hypertonia, hyperreflexia and myoclonus are commonly due to poisoning with anticholinergic compounds, sympathomimetic drugs and monoamine oxidase inhibitors. Rarely, muscle tone may be increased to such an extent that opisthotonos is present; the likely toxins then are alpha-chloralose, monoamine oxidase inhibitors and strychnine.

Anticholinergic compounds also cause extensor plantar reflexes but with deepening coma muscle tone decreases and limb and plantar reflexes may only be elicited with difficulty or not at all.

Impairment of consciousness is associated with reduced response to painful stimuli. Flexor withdrawal responses are those most commonly seen but extensor posturing also occurs. As coma becomes deeper, there may also be complete, but temporary, loss of the oculocephalic (doll's head) and oculovestibular (caloric) reflexes. Unilateral loss of the latter reflexes has been recorded in poisoned patients. Some of these changes would carry grave prognostic implications in other diseases but in acute poisoning are compatible with full and uncomplicated recovery.

Convulsions
Convulsions may be produced indirectly by hypoglycaemia and hypoxia but are more commonly due to CNS stimulation by a wide variety of chemicals, including anticholinergic compounds, sympathomimetic drugs, monoamine oxidase inhibitors, opioid analgesics, mefenamic acid and rarely salicylates, cycloserine, camphor, isoniazid and pesticides such as gamma-hexachlorocyclohexane (lindane). Paradoxically, anticonvulsants may cause convulsions when taken in excess. Patients poisoned with these substances frequently show other signs of heightened neuromuscular excitability (see above). Loud noises and painful stimuli may be sufficient to trigger convulsions.

Dystonic reactions

Dystonic reactions involving the mouth, eyes and head may be caused by metoclopramide, haloperidol, trifluperazine and prochlorperazine.

Delirium and hallucinations

Anticholinergic compounds, sympathomimetics, LSD, phencyclidine, and some mushrooms may cause delirium and hallucinations. These features are more often seen in patients recovering from the anticholinergic syndrome (p. 67) than in the early stages of poisoning. Occasionally they may be due to acute withdrawal of hypnotics or alcohol (delirium tremens).

Ocular features

Blurring of vision

Many patients complain of blurring of vision or inability to focus after overdoses of psychotropic drugs and in most they are due to generalized CNS depression. When anticholinergic drugs have been taken, difficulty in focusing is the result of paralysis of accommodation.

Loss of vision

Partial or complete loss of vision is most likely to be due to quinine or methanol.

Pupil changes

Ocular signs are common and while they are valuable diagnostic features, too much importance has been attributed in the past to pupil size and reactions. It is equally important to appreciate that other signs, such as unequal pupils and divergence of the optic axes, also occur in poisoning and are not necessarily evidence of brain damage or raised intracranial pressure.

Very small or pinpoint pupils (particularly in conjunction with a reduced respiratory rate) suggest opioid analgesic or cholinesterase inhibitor poisoning while dilated pupils are most commonly due to overdosage of drugs with anticholinergic actions (tricyclic antidepressants, antihistamines, orphenadrine, benztropine, glutethimide and thioridazine). Dilated pupils may also be seen in intoxication with LSD and sympathomimetic drugs including amphetamines, other appetite suppressants, ephedrine and theophylline and its derivatives. Occasionally, such changes are due to treatment with high-dose dopamine.

Not uncommonly, the pupils may be unequal in size while the patient is unconscious and become equal as consciousness is regained. There is no explanation for this phenomenon but its occurrence, particularly in isolation, is not a sign of rising intracranial pressure nor an indication for urgent neurosurgery.

Strabismus
Divergent strabismus, occasionally affecting the vertical as well as the horizontal axis, is frequently found in unconscious poisoned patients. It is sometimes referred to as external ophthalmoplegia or internuclear ophthalmoplegia. It occurs normally during sleep.

Papilloedema
Papilloedema is uncommon in acute poisoning and is usually due to cerebral oedema secondary to prolonged hypoxia. Carbon monoxide, methanol and glutethimide are the only poisons known to be regularly associated with papilloedema.

Nystagmus
Nystagmus is only seen in acute poisoning when the patient is sufficiently conscious to make ocular movements. It is a valuable sign of continuing intoxication and may be present when dysarthria and ataxia have largely disappeared. The nystagmus is usually rapid, fine and most easily detected on lateral gaze but in more intoxicated patients it may be rotatory, coarse and present on the slightest eye movement. Most commonly it is found during recovery from poisoning with psychotropic drugs but may also be due to phenytoin intoxication.

Subconjunctival haemorrhage
Subconjunctival haemorrhage, often extensive, may be found in young patients, especially girls. It is partly the result of raised venous pressure, particularly during vomiting and difficult gastric lavage, and partly due to the effects of salicylates on platelets and capillaries. Though there may be associated facial purpura it is uncommon to find retinal haemorrhages.

References

Greenberg DA, Simon RP. Flexor and extensor postures in sedative drug-induced coma. *Neurology* 1982; **32**: 448–451.

Kalaawi MH, Auger LT, Carroll JE *et al*. Encephalopathy and brain stem dysfunction in an infant with non-accidental carbamazepine intoxication. *Clin Pediatr* 1991; **30**: 385–386.

Nosko MG, McLean DR, Chin WDN. Loss of brainstem and pupillary reflexes in amoxapine overdose: a case report. *Clin Toxicol* 1988; **26**: 117–122.

Ong GL, Bruning HA. Dilated fixed pupils due to administration of high doses of dopamine. *Crit Care Med* 1981; **9**: 658–659.

Yang KL, Dantzker DR. Reversible brain death. A manifestation of amitriptyline overdose. *Chest* 1991; **99**: 1037–1038.

Respiratory features

Cough, sputum production, wheeze and breathlessness
Cough, sputum production, wheeze and breathlessness often occur after inhalation of irritant gases such as ammonia, chlorine, smoke from fires and the oxides of nitrogen but are more likely to be due to preexisting chronic obstructive airways disease or an aspiration pneumonia.

Cyanosis
Cyanosis in the unconscious patient is usually due to a combination of various factors including respiratory obstruction, hypoxaemia secondary to hypoventilation and ventilation–perfusion imbalance, peripheral vasoconstriction, hypotension and hypothermia. In most cases cyanosis can be abolished by attention to the airway, increasing the oxygen content of the inspired air or by assisted ventilation. Failure of these measures should suggest the possibility that the cyanosis is due to methaemoglobinaemia caused by poisons such as chlorates, nitrates, nitrites, phenol, urea herbicides (e.g. linuron and monolinuron), aniline and occasionally local anaesthetics.

Hypoventilation
Hypoventilation is common with serious overdosage with any CNS depressant and usually involves the depth of respiration. Marked reduction in respiratory rate is much less common and is usually due to intoxication with opioid analgesics.

Hyperventilation
Hyperventilation in the absence of a cardiac or respiratory cause or metabolic acidosis is most commonly due to salicylate overdosage and occasionally to CNS stimulant drugs, cyanide or phenoxyacetate herbicides.

Non-cardiogenic pulmonary oedema
Non-cardiogenic pulmonary oedema may be caused by a variety of poisons and although the mechanisms are not fully understood, it is probably due to increased pulmonary capillary permeability. Inhaled poisons (e.g. chlorine, ammonia and the oxides of nitrogen) damage the respiratory epithelium directly, as does paraquat taken orally. Ingested or injected toxins which cause pulmonary oedema include opioid analgesics (commonly seen in addicts) and salicylates.

Reference

White CD, Weiss LD. Varying presentations of methaemoglobinaemia: two cases. *J Emerg Med* 1991; **9**: 45–49.

Cardiovascular features

Loss of pulses
Loss of pulses due to peripheral circulatory failure may occur in overdosage with CNS depressants and beta-adrenoceptor blocking drugs. Rarely, it may be the result of intense arterial constriction caused by ergotamine.

Tachycardia and bradycardia
Tachycardia may be due to poisoning with anticholinergic compounds, sympathomimetic drugs and salicylates while bradycardia (other than that due to hypothermia) may be caused by cardiac glycosides, beta-adrenoceptor blocking drugs and cholinesterase inhibitors (carbamate and organophosphate insecticides).

Dysrhythmias
Dysrhythmias may be caused by a variety of drugs including cardiac glycosides, anticholinergic compounds (particularly the tricyclic anti-depressants), sympathomimetics, phenothiazines (especially thiorida-zine), chloral hydrate and antimalarials. Just as anticonvulsants may produce convulsions when taken in overdosage, many antiarrhythmic agents cause dysrhythmias when taken in excess.

Hypotension
Hypotension may occur in any severe poisoning. Central nervous system depressants commonly lower the systolic blood pressure to about 70–90 mmHg, the extent of the fall being greater with increasing depth of coma. Anticholinergic drugs are less likely to produce severe hypotension than barbiturates. These drugs and other poisons (e.g. paraquat, beta-blockers, antimalarials and iron salts) in massive doses produce hypotension by depressing myocardial contractility. Others do so by reducing the circulating blood volume through gastrointestinal loss of fluid (iron salts, mercuric chloride, strong acids and alkalis, colchicine, paraquat) or by causing venous pooling. Diuretics in overdosage produce hypotension by depleting the intravascular volume and other hypotensive drugs (bethanidine, debrisoquine and guanethi-dine) by their effect on postganglionic adrenergic nerve fibres. It must also be remembered that severe bradycardia or tachycardia may be associated with hypotension.

Hypertension
Hypertension is uncommon in acute poisoning but may be caused by sympathomimetic drugs, phencyclidine and monoamine oxidase in-hibitors. Rarely, overdosage with clonidine results in hypertension rather than hypotension.

Skin

Previous self-injury
Careful examination of the skin, notably the flexor aspects of the wrists and forearms, may yield useful evidence of previous self-injury. Scars in other areas, especially face and neck, may also have been self-inflicted while those on the chest and abdomen are more likely to have been inflicted by others.

Evidence of drug misuse
Particular attention must be paid to the skin of the arms, hands and feet. Venepuncture marks, abscesses, ulcers and thrombophlebitis usually indicate that the patient is a drug addict who has recently been mainlining. The groins should also be examined since some drug abusers, wishing to avoid having evidence of their habit where it may be seen, use the femoral vein. These findings should alert the medical and nursing staff to the potential risk of hepatitis B and human immunodeficiency virus (HIV) infection and appropriate protective measures should be taken when handling the patient, his or her blood and excreta. Unconscious addicts are likely to be poisoned with opioid analgesics or benzodiazepines, with or without ethanol.

Extensive bruising
Extensive bruising of the head, face, arms and legs suggests physical violence or the possibility of falls following intoxication with ethanol or drugs. Their presence makes it particularly important to consider skull fractures and subdural haematoma.

Purpura
Purpura, like subconjunctival haemorrhage, occurs frequently after emesis or struggling during gastric lavage. It is usually confined to the eyelids but may occasionally spread to the rest of the face and neck. Raised venous pressure, with or without the antiplatelet actions of aspirin, is usually the cause. Rarely it may be seen in young patients after protracted paroxysms of coughing following inhalation of respiratory tract irritants such as chlorine and the oxides of nitrogen. It is important to appreciate the benign nature of this form of purpura so that patients and their parents can be reassured that it will disappear in a few days and to prevent unnecessary haematological investigation.

Blistering
Patients who have lain unconscious in the same position for many hours may have erythematous areas of skin over bony prominences and pressure areas when they are found. Within a few hours of the pressure

being relieved the lesions may extend in size, become raised with a *peau d'orange* appearance, and go on to blister formation. Though they are usually found on the sides of the fingers, ankles, knees, shoulders and over the greater trochanters and iliac crests they may also form on the ears and malar region. Such blisters were formerly thought to be diagnostic of barbiturate poisoning but have now been described in association with such a wide variety of drug intoxications that they should be regarded as non-specific.

Sweating
Salicylate overdosage is the likeliest explanation for excessive sweating after poisoning but infection and hypoglycaemia should be sought and treated if present. Less commonly, it is due to phencyclidine or organophosphates.

Urinary features

Urinary symptoms are seldom encountered after poisoning. Retention of urine is common after overdosage with anticholinergic drugs but the patients are usually unconscious or too drowsy to complain of difficulty in micturating; incontinence is often the first clue in patients whose abdomens are not examined sufficiently frequently. Anuria is usually due to acute tubular necrosis and may be caused by numerous poisons. Polyuria occurs during recovery from tubular necrosis or may be due to lithium-induced diabetes insipidus.

Auditory symptoms

Tinnitus and deafness are common complaints after salicylate poisoning and are present in virtually every adult whose plasma salicylate concentration exceeds 300 mg/l (2.2 mmol/l). These symptoms also occur after quinine poisoning but this is comparatively uncommon.

Temperature disturbances

Hypothermia
Hypothermia (rectal temperature <35°C) commonly occurs after overdosage with CNS depressant drugs, especially alcohol and phenothiazines, and its incidence increases with increasing depth of coma. Environmental temperature is obviously important, but severe hypothermia can occur even in summer. Body temperature usually increases spontaneously as consciousness is regained and during recovery it may rise above normal in the absence of infection or tissue necrosis. Fever is not in itself an indication for antibiotics.

Hyperthermia

Hyperthermia may complicate poisoning with substances which uncouple oxidative phosphorylation (usually salicylates), have anticholinergic effects or cause a generalized increase in neuromuscular activity (sympathomimetic drugs and monoamine oxidase inhibitors).

Hyperthermia due to salicylates and anticholinergic drugs is more common in childhood than adult poisoning.

Diagnostic trials of antidotes

In patients who are unconscious for reasons which are not known, it may be possible to reach a diagnosis of poisoning by trial administration of an antidote. It is essential in such circumstances that the antidote itself carries minimal hazards and this limits those that can be used in this way. The antidotes likely to produce the most dramatic responses are naloxone and flumazenil which may completely reverse coma and the associated consequences of CNS depression within 1–2 minutes. Their use is described on pages 164 and 81 respectively. Clearly, the value of diagnostic trials of naloxone will depend on the prevalence of misuse of opioid analgesics in the community in which it is being used. A recent study from Pittsburgh, USA, of blind administration of 0.4–0.8 mg by paramedics to a large number of patients with acute loss of consciousness resulted in total or partial improvement only in about 11%. There were no serious safety concerns.

Desferrioxamine may also be used as a diagnostic agent (see p. 137).

References

Burkhart KK, Kulig KW. The diagnostic utility of flumazenil (a benzodiazepine antagonist) in coma of unknown etiology. *Ann Emerg Med* 1990; **19**: 319–321.
Yealy DM, Paris PM, Kaplan RM *et al*. The safety of prehospital naloxone administration by paramedics. *Ann Emerg Med* 1990; **19**: 902–905.

Exclusion of other causes of coma

General considerations

When the history and circumstantial evidence strongly suggest that coma is due to poisoning there is generally little need for more than a careful physical examination to exclude other causes. Sometimes, however, the diagnosis of poisoning may be considerably less secure and care must be exercised in excluding other pathology. Further assessment must be guided by the philosophy that it is unforgivable to miss conditions which are treatable.

The differential diagnosis of coma is extremely wide and detailed discussion here would be inappropriate. Fortunately many conditions, including meningitis, trauma, hypoglycaemia, diabetic ketoacidosis, uraemia, hepatic encephalopathy and most cerebrovascular accidents, are unlikely to be confused with poisoning by an experienced clinician. On the other hand encephalitis, subarachnoid haemorrhage, brainstem vascular lesions and subdural and extradural haematomas can cause diagnostic difficulties. Suspicion that coma is not the result of poisoning may be aroused by features in the history, physical examination and by the clinical course during the first few hours after admission to hospital.

History

A history of premonitory headache, behaviour changes, nausea and vomiting for a few hours or days before becoming unconscious strongly suggests the presence of an aneurysm, encephalitis or mass lesion within the skull, particularly if there also have been focal neurological symptoms. Any possibility of recent head injury should stimulate a search for evidence of traumatic intracranial haemorrhage.

Examination

Abrasions and lacerations
Abrasions and lacerations of the scalp increase the possibility of a subdural or extradural haemorrhage, especially if there is bleeding from the ears or nose. Extensive bruising of the limbs and trunk may also be associated with these diagnoses since falls in individuals chronically intoxicated with alcohol or psychotropic drugs can lead to intracranial damage.

Inequality of pupil size
Inequality of the pupils is usually considered to be a particularly ominous sign but, found in isolation, is not necessarily an indication of rising intracranial pressure as it may be due to a Holmes–Adie pupil or instillation of drugs into the conjunctival sac.

Lateralizing neurological signs
Lateralizing neurological signs are strongly against a diagnosis of poisoning unless they can be explained by some previous illness, e.g. a cerebrovascular accident. Unfortunately, brainstem vascular lesions and subarachnoid haemorrhage may be sufficiently severe to make the

patient deeply unconscious without lateralizing signs and with hypo-reflexia and absent plantar responses. In such cases suspicion may be first aroused when the patient fails to progress as would be expected if poisoning were the cause of coma.

Papilloedema
Papilloedema is not a feature of poisoning other than with glutethimide or carbon monoxide unless cerebral oedema has developed following prolonged hypoxia or hypotension.

Clinical course

The great majority of patients with drug-induced coma show significant improvement in conscious level within 12 hours of admission to hospital. Some, particularly with phenobarbitone, meprobamate or ethchlorvynol poisoning, require longer (24–48 hours) and a few may become more deeply unconscious before improving. However, such cases are sufficiently uncommon that failure to improve within 12 hours should raise the possibility of some other cause for coma. Rapid deterioration in consciousness with the development of unilateral pupillary dilatation or respiratory arrest is much more likely to be due to some intracranial lesion than to poisoning.

Measures to take

Once the clinical suspicion has been raised that coma is not due to drugs various steps should be taken:

1 Interview the patient's relatives and reappraise the history.
2 Reexamine the patient frequently with particular attention to the neurological system. Repeat fundoscopy looking for signs of early papilloedema or subhyaloid haemorrhage. The optic fundi may be difficult to visualize in many cases if the pupils are small or if central cataracts are present, but with skill and perseverance the optic discs can usually be seen. Never use mydriatics to facilitate retinoscopy as this deprives the clinician of the diagnostic value of spontaneous dilatation of one pupil. The scalp should also be reexamined and the soft tissues in the temporal fossae compared since unilateral swelling may be the result of trauma with a possible skull fracture and extradural haematoma.
3 Measure the blood or plasma glucose concentration if it has not already be done.
4 Skull radiography excludes fractures and shows pineal displacement or, rarely, calcification in an arteriovenous malformation.

5 Obtain a computed tomography scan of the head.
6 Send urine and plasma to the laboratory to be screened for drugs. The limitations of this approach are discussed on p. 23.

Laboratory investigations

Haematological and biochemical investigations are often performed on the poisoned patient who is seriously ill. The results may suggest possible poisons in cases where there is doubt about the exact nature of the compound involved, but it must be emphasized that abnormal results are not of direct diagnostic significance.

Examination of urine

Changes in the colour of the urine occasionally occur as a result of acute poisoning.

1 Green or blue urine occurs when proprietary preparations containing methylene blue are taken.
2 Orange or orange-red urine is found with overdosage of rifampicin or after treatment of iron poisoning with desferrioxamine.
3 Urine which is grey to black in colour strongly suggests poisoning with compounds containing phenols and cresols, e.g. Lysol, and may be confirmed by their characteristic smell.
4 Primidone may crystallize in the urine as it cools. If the urine is then shaken whorls of shimmering, highly refractile crystals can be seen. On microscopy each crystal can be seen to be a needle-shaped hexagon. Their chemical nature is readily confirmed by simple analytical techniques.
5 Brown discoloration may be due to the presence of paracetamol metabolites or haemoglobin or myoglobin if there is intravascular haemolysis or rhabdomyolysis.

Inspection of blood and plasma

Arterialization of venous blood (i.e. an unexpected red colour) may suggest poisoning with cyanides while freshly drawn venous blood that is chocolate-brown in colour suggests methaemoglobinaemia and poisoning with oxidizing agents such as chlorates, aniline, nitrates, nitrites, dapsone, local anaesthetics, some urea herbicides or nomifensine.

Pink or brown discoloration of plasma, assuming the blood sample was taken with care, suggests haemolysis and possible poisoning with chlorates, dapsone, nomifensine, urea herbicides or arsine.

Haematological investigations

Haematological investigations are of very little help in suggesting specific poisons or groups of poisons. The white cell count is often raised in acute poisoning, probably due to tissue necrosis. Leucopenia and thrombocytopenia may complicate overdosage with cytotoxic agents. In severe poisoning, isolated thrombocytopenia is more likely to be due to disseminated intravascular coagulation.

Prothrombin time prolongation may be caused by ingestion of anticoagulants such as warfarin and superwarfarins or secondary to severe liver necrosis induced by paracetamol, iron salts, some mushrooms, carbon tetrachloride, isoniazid and phenylbutazone.

Biochemical findings

Hyperkalaemia

Hyperkalaemia in acute poisoning may be due to potassium overload (ingestion or therapeutic administration of potassium salts), impaired excretion (renal failure), liberation from damaged tissues (as in rhabdomyolysis), shift from the intracellular to the extracellular compartment caused by the actions of the poison on the cell membrane sodium/potassium pump or secondary to metabolic acidosis. Commonly, two or more of these causes may operate in individual patients. Table 2.1 lists poisons which alter plasma potassium concentrations.

Hypokalaemia

Hypokalaemia in acute poisoning is usually the result of redistribution from the extracellular to the intracellular compartment secondary to stimulation of the cell membrane sodium/potassium pump by the poison. The toxins with which hypokalaemia has been associated are listed in Table 2.1.

Hypocalcaemia

Hypocalcaemia is commonly due to chelation of plasma calcium by fluorides, oxalic acid (usually from metabolism of ethylene glycol) or phosphates. It has also been reported in overdosage with calcium channel blockers and during attempts to induce an alkaline diuresis.

Reduced plasma bicarbonate

Reduction of the plasma bicarbonate concentration in the early stages of acute poisoning is most likely to be due to the presence of a metabolic acidosis and, unless severe, is of little diagnostic value. It is more important as an indication to carry out arterial blood gas analysis for more accurate assessment.

Table 2.1 Toxins which alter plasma K⁺ through effects on cell membrane sodium/ potassium pumps

Hyperkalaemia	Hypokalaemia
Atenolol	Barium carbonate
Digitalis	Barium chloride
Digitoxin	Caffeine
Digoxin	Chloroquine
Disopyramide	Disopyramide
Fluoride salts	Ethylene glycol butyl ether
Ibuprofen	Insulin
Opioid analgesics	Magnesium sulphate
Oxprenolol	Nalidixic acid
Potassium chloride	Nifedipine
	Oxpentifylline
	Quinine
	Salbutamol
	Sotalol
	Terbutaline
	Theophylline
	Toluene
	Yew leaves
	Zimeldine

When reduction of the plasma bicarbonate is marked, a high anion gap acidosis may be present and the result is of greater diagnostic usefulness. The anion gap is calculated from the equation:

Anion gap = $[Na] - ([Cl] + [HCO_3])$

The anion gap is normally 12 ± 2 and increases indicate a metabolic acidosis. The poisons which commonly cause a high anion gap acidosis include ethanol, methanol, ethylene glycol, cyanide, isoniazid, salicylates and strychnine. This list may be further reduced by also measuring the osmolal gap (p. 121).

Less commonly, reduction of the plasma bicarbonate may be the result of respiratory alkalosis as in intoxication with salicylates, sympathomimetic agents, LSD and phenoxyacetate herbicides.

Hyperglycaemia
Poisoning with the substances listed in Table 2.2 has been reported to cause hyperglycaemia. The explanation for this abnormality is not always clear. Occasionally it complicates massive liver necrosis.

Hypoglycaemia
Hypoglycaemia in acute poisoning may be due to the direct effects of toxins such as ethanol, insulin, oral hypoglycaemic agents,

Table 2.2 Toxins which have been reported to cause hyperglycaemia

Acetone	Nifedipine
Adrenaline	Phenylbutazone
Cadmium chloride	Phenylpropanolamine
Caffeine	Salicylates
Clonidine	Sodium azide
Cyanide	Terbutaline
Iron salts	Theophylline
Isoniazid	Verapamil
Isopropanol	Water hemlock
Methanol	Yew leaves
Nalidixic acid	Zinc chloride

beta-adrenoceptor blockers and salicylates. It may also be secondary to massive hepatic necrosis caused by substances such as paracetamol, some mushrooms, carbon tetrachloride, iron salts, isoniazid and phenylbutazone.

Screening for poisons

The purpose of an emergency laboratory drug screen is to identify and quantify poisons amenable to specific treatment in patients who are desperately ill and in whom the exact nature of the poison is uncertain. It should not be used merely to confirm the diagnosis suspected from the history or circumstantial evidence unless a positive result will alter management; all the evidence indicates that it is of limited value. Laboratory screens for poisons are tedious and time-consuming and require considerable expertise. They should not be used as an alternative to detailed questioning of the relatives, ambulance crew and family doctor to find out which drugs were available or to a thorough search for and interpretation of abnormal physical signs.

The only indiscriminate screening which can be justified despite a low positivity rate is the search for paracetamol in unconscious overdose patients (see p. 44).

No laboratory screen can be expected to detect all possible poisons and the clinical chemist requires as much guidance as the clinician can provide to help direct the analyses. It is therefore essential that requests for drug screens should be discussed beforehand by the clinician and the laboratory staff. Remember that laboratory staff engaged in prolonged and pointless drug screens cannot at the same time be expected to provide the urgent and much more useful clinical chemistry service often necessary for the management of severely poisoned patients.

When a drug screen is requested the laboratory should be provided with samples of gastric aspirate and urine as well as blood. Drugs and their metabolites are usually present in aspirate and urine in much higher concentrations than in blood, and urine usually has the advantage of being available in larger volumes. Although the urine may be used for identification of the poisons, only their concentrations in plasma or blood are useful for management and prognosis.

References

Ashbourne JF, Olson KR, Khayam-Bashi H. Value of rapid screening for acetaminophen in all patients with intentional drug overdose. *Ann Emerg Med* 1990; **18**: 1035–1038.

Jammehdiabadi M, Tierney M. Impact of toxicology screens in the diagnosis of a suspected overdose: salicylates, tricyclic antidepressants, and benzodiazepines. *Vet Hum Toxicol* 1991; **33**: 40–43.

Kellermann AL, Fihn SD, LoGerfo JP *et al.* Impact of drug screening in suspected overdose. *Ann Emerg Med* 1987; **16**: 1206–1216.

Mahoney JD, Gross PL, Stern TA *et al.* Quantitative serum toxic screening in the management of suspected drug overdose. *Am J Emerg Med* 1990; **8**: 16–22.

Wiley JF. Difficult diagnoses in toxicology. Poisons not detected by the comprehensive drug screen. *Pediatr Clin North Am* 1991; **38**: 725–737.

Electrocardiography

Since drugs with prominent anticholinergic actions are amongst the most common taken in overdosage, electrocardiographic findings may suggest poisoning as a cause of otherwise unexplained coma. The changes are detailed under amitriptyline (p. 66). The well-documented electrocardiogram changes of overdosage with cardiac glycosides (p. 114) may also be identified.

Reference

Niemann JT, Bessen HA, Rothstein RJ *et al.* Electrocardiographic criteria for tricyclic antidepressant cardiotoxicity. *Am J Cardiol* 1986; **57**: 1154–1159.

Radiology

Radiology is of very limited diagnostic value in acute poisoning. While it is invaluable in confirming ingestion of metallic objects such as button batteries, only a very small proportion of pharmaceutical preparations are radiopaque. Iron and sustained-release potassium tablets may be visible on an abdominal radiograph and it may also be possible to confirm the ingestion of petroleum distillates on an abdominal film taken in the erect position. The hydrocarbon forms a faintly radiopaque layer between normal gastric contents and the gas above.

A chest radiograph showing pulmonary oedema in a poisoned patient suggests overdosage with opioid analgesics, salicylates or ethchlorvynol. Similar appearances may be found after inhalation of gases such as chlorine or the oxides of nitrogen, but in these cases the interval between poisoning and development of pulmonary oedema is measured in hours rather than in minutes.

Reference

O'Brien RP, McGeehan PA, Helmeczi AW *et al*. Detectability of drug tablets and capsules by plain radiography. *Am J Emerg Med* 1986; **4**: 302–312.

Points of emphasis

- Diagnosis of poisoning is made from the history and circumstantial evidence in the majority of cases.
- Patients' statements about the nature and quantity of drugs ingested must be accepted with caution.
- Poisoning is one of the most common causes of non-traumatic coma in patients under the age of 35 years.
- Isolated symptoms and signs are of no diagnostic value.
- Constellations of symptoms and signs are of diagnostic value.
- Organic brain damage should be suspected if the history of poisoning is unsatisfactory and the depth of coma does not improve within 12 hours.
- Routine biochemical and haematological investigations may rarely suggest a diagnosis of acute poisoning.
- Screening of all unconscious poisoned patients for paracetamol is justified.
- Requests for drug screens should always be discussed with laboratory staff.
- Gastric aspirate and urine are often more useful for drug screens than blood or plasma.
- Abdominal radiographs may occasionally reveal evidence of ingestion of iron and potassium preparations.

Chapter 3

General plan for the management of acute poisoning

The severity of physical illness following acute poisoning varies widely. About 90% of children and adults have minimal symptoms and require correspondingly little medical care. On the other hand, at least half of the remainder are very seriously ill and their recovery depends on the highest standards of medical and nursing care. The majority of them have taken central nervous system (CNS) depressant drugs and management of coma is a vital part of the general approach to the treatment of poisoning. The following steps should be implemented according to the patient's condition:

1 Ensure that the airway, ventilation and blood pressure are adequate.
2 Assess the level of consciousness.
3 Contact the poisons information services if there is uncertainty about the toxicity of the substance or the management of poisoning with it.
4 Consider whether an antidote is available, appropriate or necessary.
5 Consider the need for measures to prevent absorption of the poison.
6 Consider whether an emergency drug analysis should be requested.
7 Institute a programme of continuing care.
8 Consider whether it is possible or desirable to attempt to increase the elimination of the poison.

Maintenance of vital functions

In any severely poisoned patient the first priorities are to ensure that the airway is clear and that alveolar ventilation and cardiac output are adequate to maintain life while decisions are being made about further treatment. Although these functions are considered separately, it must be emphasized that they are interdependent.

Airway

Upper airway obstruction is one of the most common causes of death in patients dying from poisoning outside hospital. The establishment of a clear airway automatically improves alveolar ventilation and often restores blood pressure but will not affect coexisting central respiratory depression.

1 Remove dental plates, making sure that they are carefully set aside and later labelled and stored for return to the patient when consciousness is regained.
2 Use the chin-lift and jaw-thrust manoeuvres to clear an airway obstructed by the tongue falling back.
3 Remove saliva or vomitus from the mouth and pharynx. Ideally this is best achieved using a suction catheter, but in an emergency a swab wrapped round a finger is highly effective. When suction is used it is important to avoid inducing gagging and vomiting. Avoid passing catheters through the nose since trauma to the highly vascular nasal epithelium may cause profuse bleeding and add to the difficulties of keeping the airway clear. However, prior insertion of a soft nasopharyngeal airway would protect the epithelium.
4 Insert an endotracheal tube if the patient is deeply unconscious and the cough reflex is depressed or absent. Adult males and females require tubes of 9.0–9.5 mm diameter and 8.0–8.5 mm respectively. The internal diameter (mm) of tube required for children aged 4–12 years is calculated by the formula:

$$\frac{Age\ (years)}{4} + 4.5$$

The size of the tube does not matter when the patient is being mechanically ventilated but is important during spontaneous ventilation when respiratory effort is increased by a tube that is too small.
5 Ensure that the tube has not been inserted too far since it may enter the right main bronchus, obstruct the left main bronchus and cause atelectasis of the left lung. This can be avoided if care is taken to use a tube which is not too long and by auscultating the lungs immediately after intubation to check that there is air entry into both sides. A chest X-ray should always be taken and will ideally show the tip of the tube above the carina, level with the medial ends of the clavicles.
6 Insert a short oropharyngeal airway if the patient is unconscious but unable to accept or tolerate an endotracheal tube. A size 3 airway is suitable for most small or medium-height adults but some may

require a size 4. Alternatively, a soft nasopharyngeal tube may be used.

7 Turn the patient into the semiprone or three-quarters prone position unless an endotracheal tube has been inserted, in which case the supine position is acceptable. If an oropharyngeal tube is being used keep the neck flexed and the head extended with the lower jaw pulled forward to increase the anteroposterior diameter of the larynx.

Ventilation

Emergency measures

The most important aspect of improving ventilation is to establish a clear airway as described above. Once this has been done, however, the rate and/or depth of respiration may still be inadequate and immediate steps must be taken to remedy this situation. Outside hospital, start mouth-to-mouth respiration or assist ventilation with whatever suitable equipment is to hand. In hospital use an Ambu bag or similar apparatus via a face mask or endotracheal tube; do not wait for the results of arterial blood gas analysis. Oxygen should be given and naloxone administered if there is any suspicion of overdosage with an opioid analgesic (see p. 164 for dosage).

Assessment of ventilation

In less urgent circumstances the adequacy of ventilation is best assessed by arterial blood gas analysis. This vital investigation is only as valuable as the care taken in obtaining the sample and assessing the results. Attention should be given to the following details:

1 Ensure at the time of sampling that the blood is arterial and not venous. The only certain way to decide this is to observe the blood pulsating into the syringe. Contrary to popular belief, the origin of the blood cannot be determined from its colour or the results of analysis. Unfortunately the more ill the patient, the greater the difficulty in obtaining an arterial sample and the more crucial the investigation.

2 If using a syringe which is individually packed and already heparinized, be sure to squirt out the excess heparin before taking the sample. If using an ordinary syringe, use the correct concentration of heparin and use as little as possible. A concentration of 1000 iu/ml is satisfactory and the quantity required to fill the needle and hub of the syringe is more than enough. Excessive quantities significantly alter blood gas tensions and raise the hydrogen ion concentration.

3 Obtain a minimum sample volume of 3 ml to reduce interference from heparin and air bubbles.

Measurement of respiratory minute volume by some type of spirometer (e.g. a Wright spirometer) is of limited value in the assessment of the adequacy of ventilation and has been largely superseded by the ready availability of arterial blood gas analysis in most hospitals. Note that it is no longer considered justified to correct arterial blood gas tensions for body core temperature.

Ventilation and acid–base disturbances in coma
Patients who are unconscious after overdoses of barbiturates or tricyclic antidepressants, but still self-ventilating, seldom show marked carbon dioxide retention though the PaCO$_2$ is often near the upper limit of normal. However, the arterial oxygen tension may be unexpectedly low, particularly in grade 4 coma and to a lesser extent in grade 3 coma, probably due to ventilation/perfusion imbalance (see p. 30 for definition of coma grades). The consequence of combined hypoxia and mild carbon dioxide retention is a rise in arterial hydrogen ion concentration (reduction of pH) due to a mixed metabolic and respiratory acidosis. Under no circumstance should attempts be made to correct the metabolic component of the acid–base disturbance by infusion of alkali before the PaCO$_2$ has been brought within the normal range. Hypoxia can usually be corrected by increasing the oxygen content of inspired air.

Interpretation of the results of arterial blood gas analysis and monitoring of the effects of corrective measures are most readily achieved by plotting them on an acid–base diagram.

Improving ventilation
Establishment of a clear airway is of paramount importance in improving ventilation. In the deeply unconscious adult endotracheal intubation reduces the respiratory physiological dead space by about 60–70 ml and increases alveolar ventilation correspondingly. If ventilation remains inadequate despite these measures, assisted respiration is necessary. The type of ventilator used will depend on what is available and is best chosen in conjunction with anaesthetists.

Reference

Sutherland GR, Park J, Proudfoot AT. Ventilation and acid–base changes in deep coma due to barbiturate or tricyclic antidepressant poisoning. *Clin Toxicol* 1977; **11**: 403–412.

Hypotension

It is difficult to define hypotension in acute poisoning. By custom the minimum acceptable systolic blood pressure readings are 80 mmHg in young adults and 90 mmHg in patients aged more than 40 years.

However, these values are arbitrary and more reliance should be placed on organ perfusion as assessed by the patient's mental state (if conscious), skin temperature or hourly urine output (if catheterized). When hypotension is a problem:

1 Identify the probable cause or causes (see p. 14).
2 Clear the airway, improve ventilation and correct hypoxia – this will abolish hypotension in many unconscious patients.
3 Correct any metabolic acidosis which persists after hypoxia and hypercapnia have been abolished.
4 Insert a central venous line if the patient fails to respond to the above measures.
5 If the central venous pressure (CVP) is low expand the intravascular volume with plasma or plasma substitute.
6 Give dopamine (2–10 μg/kg per min intravenously) if the CVP is high or expanding the intravascular volume is ineffective.
7 Rarely, hypotension may remain a serious problem despite these measures and may only improve when some procedure is instituted to remove poison from the circulation (e.g. charcoal haemoperfusion).

Assessment of the level of consciousness

Various methods of grading the level of consciousness of poisoned patients are in use. The Edinburgh method is recommended because it is simple and the grades of coma defined correlate with other features of poisoning, including the presence of hypotension, hypothermia and depression of the cough reflex and respiration. Classification is based on the response to commands and pain.

Grade 0: Fully conscious.
Grade 1: Drowsy but obeys commands.
Grade 2: Unresponsive to commands but responds well to pain.
Grade 3: Unresponsive to commands and minimally responsive to pain.
Grade 4: Completely unresponsive.

Squeezing the rim of the ear is an adequate painful stimulus. Rubbing the sternum with the knuckles is not advised since frequent repetition soon leads to bruising and oedema. By definition, patients in grades 2, 3 and 4 are unconscious. Assessment of level of consciousness should be delayed until the airway and ventilation are satisfactory. The Glasgow coma score is also widely used to monitor changes in poisoned patients, although it has not been validated for this purpose.

Reference

Starmark JE, Heath A. Severity grading in acute poisoning. *Hum Toxicol* 1988; **7**: 551–555.

Poisons information services

No doctor is expected to know the constituents of the infinite array of drugs, household products and agricultural and industrial preparations that may be involved in poisoning episodes, far less their toxic effects and appropriate treatment. Poisons information services were established to provide such information and any doctor dealing with a poisoned patient is strongly advised to contact the nearest centre if he or she is in any doubt about the nature or toxicity and the best treatment for the particular poison. The telephone numbers of the UK centres are given in Appendix 1 (p. 232). If maximum benefit is to be obtained from an enquiry it is important to appreciate the limitations of these services.

1 An enquiry may initially be answered by a nurse, secretary, pharmacist, information scientist or doctor, none of whom necessarily has special knowledge or clinical experience of poisoning. They will consult the appropriate entry in their database and read out the relevant constituents and toxic effects of the poison and the recommended treatment. Inevitably, the amount of information given is often limited and general in nature, and if it does not meet the needs, the enquirer should not hesitate to ask to speak to medical staff with practical experience of poisoning.
2 Make certain that you and the person answering the call are in no doubt about the correct spelling of the name of the poison or product. Failure to do so may prevent available information being found or result in misleading and potentially dangerous advice being given.
3 Give the brand name of the drug or commercial product whenever possible. There may be more than one toxic ingredient and you may not necessarily identify the most important one from the list of constituents. Moreover the concentration of the same toxin in different products may vary from insignificant to potentially very dangerous.
4 If you do not know the precise name of the poison but know its purpose (e.g. drain cleaner, dry cleaning agent, bleach, etc.), an enquiry in these general terms may still be worthwhile.
5 Do not be dismayed if information about the poison is sketchy or not available, as is frequently the case with uncommon chemicals and industrial compounds. The lack of information simply reflects the rarity of poisoning.

6 Do not expect poisons information services to identify plants and mushrooms from descriptions given over the telephone. These must be identified by the enquirer.

7 Do not ask patients or their relatives to telephone the poisons information centre. It is policy in the UK to give information only to medically qualified enquirers since telling an already worried patient or parent the features of poisoning might only increase anxiety. It is also arguable that only doctors can assess the seriousness of poisoning and the need for treatment.

8 Beware of acting on information obtained through middle parties. The more serious the poisoning episode, the more important it is for the doctor involved personally to ask for advice. Do not leave this task to nurses, secretaries or pharmacists who are not trained to discuss clinical complexities or the relative merits of different forms of treatment.

9 Please answer any request from the information service for details of the course and outcome of a poisoning you have managed. This may be the only way that knowledge of poisoning with new or uncommon compounds can be obtained.

It must be emphasized that poisons information centres exist to provide information and advice, not to make decisions for the doctor managing the patient. Only that doctor is in a position to assess fully the clinical situation and decide what action is most appropriate.

Antidotes

The administration of antidotes to certain poisons can occasionally produce dramatic and life-saving improvement in a patient's condition and obviate the need for protracted intensive care. However, contrary to popular belief, antidotes are available for only a very small number of poisons, most of which are uncommon in everyday clinical practice. They are listed with their appropriate antidotes in Table 3.1 together with the mode of action of the antidotes. Details about use are given under the specific poisons.

Preventing absorption

Poisons may be absorbed from the respiratory tract, skin, gastro-intestinal tract or combinations of these. Body packing poses special problems.

Table 3.1 Antidotes

Poisons	Antidote	Mode of action
Anticholinergic compounds	Physostigmine salicylate	Cholinesterase inhibitor
Anticoagulants (oral)	Vitamin K$^+$ Fresh frozen plasma Clotting factors	Pharmacological antagonist Replacement of missing clotting factors
Beta-adrenoceptor blockers	Isoprenaline Glucagon	Pharmacological antagonist Stimulates myocardial adenocyclase
Cyanide	Dicobalt edetate	Chelating agent
Ethylene glycol	Ethanol	Competitive substrate for alcohol dehydrogenase
Heavy metals	Dimercaprol Penicillamine	Chelating agents
Iron salts	Desferrioxamine	Chelating agent
Methanol	Ethanol	Competitive substrate for alcohol dehydrogenase
Opioid analgesics	Naloxone	Pharmacological antagonist
Organophosphate insecticides	Atropine Pralidoxime	Acetylcholine antagonist Cholinesterase reactivator
Paracetamol	N-acetylcysteine Methionine	Glutathione precursors
Pentazocine	Naloxone	Pharmacological antagonist
Sympathomimetics	Beta-adrenoceptor blockers	Pharmacological antagonist
Thallium	Prussian blue	Chelating agent

Inhaled poisons

Removal of victims from toxic atmospheres is the function of rescue services and is unlikely to fall to medical staff. However, the possibility of continued inhalation of potential poisons from contaminated clothing must be remembered and appropriate action instituted at an early stage. Rescuers must take precautions to avoid becoming contaminated themselves (e.g. by wearing gloves, gowns and breathing apparatus, as indicated by the physicochemical properties and routes of absorption of the toxin).

Poisons contaminating the skin

The importance of decontaminating skin which has been soiled by poisons is self-evident. The patient's clothing must be removed and the skin thoroughly washed with soap and warm water. Time should not be wasted waiting for skin applications which are said to have specific value; with the exception of calcium gluconate gel for hydrofluoric acid burns, most have none. Again, rescuers must take precautions to avoid becoming contaminated themselves.

Ingested poisons

When a toxin has been ingested it would seem logical to attempt to minimize its absorption. There are three ways in which this might be achieved: by emptying the stomach, administration of activated charcoal and whole-bowel irrigation.

Is it useful to try to empty the stomach?
Unfortunately, however sound the theory, there is considerable controversy over the value of gastric emptying. It has been appreciated for some years that gastric lavage is carried out much too often, usually by nurses on the instructions of junior doctors who, doubting the veracity of patients' statements about what was swallowed and generally without too much thought about what it is hoped to achieve, believe the procedure to be in the interests of safety. For similar reasons, induced emesis is employed far too frequently; its convenience for staff and the very high incidence of vomiting it achieves (both in children and adults) encourage abuse. Clinical toxicologists have not helped by failing to provide sufficiently clear indications for gastric emptying. The current evidence indicates that:

1 Controlled trials indicate that gastric emptying does not significantly alter the course of poisoning.
2 Toxicologically important quantities of drugs are recovered in only a very small minority of those subjected to gastric emptying procedures. In most, less than two therapeutic doses are retrieved.
3 Large quantities of drug have been found in the upper alimentary tract at post-mortem or endoscopy despite apparently successful emptying of the stomach. In some of these cases too small a tube may have been used or the drug had formed a large concretion.
4 Gastric lavage may increase the severity of poisoning by forcing toxin through the pylorus and enhancing its absorption.
5 Hypoxia is not uncommon during gastric lavage and may predispose to the development of dysrhythmias when cardiotoxic agents have been taken.
6 Ipecacuanha administration is not as harmless as many would like to believe. Vomiting may persist long beyond the period when poison

might be ejected and delay administration of charcoal which might be more beneficial. Lethargy, drowsiness and diarrhoea occur in up to 13% of cases and aspiration in about 5%. More serious complications including Mallory–Weiss syndrome and gastric rupture are fortunately rare.

As a result, there is an undoubted trend towards abandoning gastric lavage and induced emesis in the management of mild and moderate poisoning and replacing them with repeated doses of oral activated charcoal, the reasoning being that the amounts of drug retrieved could more easily be adsorbed by charcoal (see p. 40).

References

Garrettson LK. Ipecac home use: we need hope replaced with data. *J Toxicol Clin Toxicol* 1991; **29**: 515–519.

Jorens PG, Joosens EJ, Nagler JM. Changes in arterial oxygen tension after gastric lavage for drug overdose. *Hum Exp Toxicol* 1991; **10**: 221–224.

Kornberg AE, Dolgin J. Pediatric ingestions: charcoal alone versus ipecac and charcoal. *Ann Emerg Med* 1991; **20**: 648–651.

Merigian KS, Woodward M, Hedges JR *et al*. Prospective evaluation of gastric emptying in the self-poisoned patient. *Am J Emerg Med* 1990; **8**: 479–483.

Saetta JP, Quinton DN. Residual gastric content after gastric lavage and ipecacuanha-induced emesis in self-poisoned patients: an endoscopic study. *J R Soc Med* 1991; **84**: 35–38.

Saetta JP, March S, Gaunt ME *et al*. Gastric emptying procedures in the self-poisoned patient: are we forcing gastric content beyond the pylorus? *J R Soc Med* 1991; **84**: 274–276.

Vale JA, Meredith TJ, Proudfoot AT. Syrup of ipecacuanha: is it really useful? *Br Med J* 1986; **293**: 1321–1322.

Wason S. Gastrointestinal decontamination of the poisoned patient - a critical review. *Drugs Today* 1987; **23**: 455–465.

When to empty the stomach

The dilemma of identifying the patients most likely to benefit from gastric emptying is unlikely ever to be resolved and hard-and-fast rules cannot be laid down. Instead, make a decision after considering the following:

1 *Has a dangerous compound been ingested?* It is obvious that the more toxic the poison, the more important it is to retrieve any remaining in the stomach. In contrast, relatively innocuous compounds (e.g. oral contraceptive preparations, benzodiazepines) make it less necessary to empty the stomach.

2 *Has a dangerous quantity been ingested?* Some poisons (e.g. cyanide and some formulations of paraquat) are potentially lethal even in very small quantities and it would seem wise to empty the stomach. However, some of the dangers of lavage noted above (especially

point 4) may make the procedure counterproductive; there are no data on which to make rational decisions. Other poisons have to be taken in large amounts before they are likely to be dangerous. Danger has to be assessed, not only in terms of life or death, but also in terms of the severity and duration of toxic effects. The amount likely to be dangerous will clearly vary according to the weight of the patient. Assessment of the risk may require considerable experience.

3 *How long since ingestion?* The time since ingestion is important in determining how much drug is likely to be in the stomach and available for recovery. The rate at which the stomach empties is increased by previous gastric surgery and delayed when the patient is unconscious. However in most circumstances there is unlikely to be benefit in emptying the stomach if longer than 2 hours has elapsed since ingestion.

4 *Has the poison altered the rate of gastric emptying?* The poison itself can reduce or accelerate the rate of gastric emptying. Drugs such as metoclopramide and irritant poisons such as paraquat probably increase the rate of gastric emptying while anticholinergic compounds and opioid analgesics delay emptying and increase the time during which gastric emptying may be beneficial. Even with the latter, however, there is probably nothing to be gained from emptying the stomach after 6 hours have elapsed since ingestion. It has been suggested that salicylates cause pyloric spasm and that significant quantities may be retrieved up to 24 hours from ingestion but the evidence is unconvincing and the same guidelines probably apply to salicylates as to other drugs.

5 *Is the patient unconscious?* The presence of coma is usually a reliable indicator that a large amount of toxin has been ingested and absorbed. As coma becomes deeper bowel sounds tend to disappear and it is assumed that gastric emptying is delayed as part of the overall reduction in gut activity. It is therefore recommended that gastric aspiration and lavage be carried out in every unconscious poisoned patient if the airway can be protected.

When NOT to empty the stomach

1 *The airway cannot be protected.* Emptying the stomach, whether by inducing emesis or by lavage tube, is only safe if the respiratory passages can be protected. The patient therefore must have an adequate cough reflex or be sufficiently depressed that a cuffed endotracheal tube can be inserted. To persist with gastric lavage in a patient who cannot cough adequately yet is too 'light' to accept an endotracheal tube is to invite acute respiratory obstruction or aspiration pneumonia. In such cases the help of an anaesthetist should be sought and an endotracheal tube inserted before proceeding.

2 *A petroleum distillate has been taken.* Petroleum distillates (long chain hydrocarbons) can cause serious pneumonia if aspirated into the lungs. Unless large enough amounts have been ingested it is customary to recommend that gastric emptying, by any method, should be avoided (p. 192).

3 *A corrosive substance has been swallowed.* Ingestion of corrosives agents is a contraindication to emptying the stomach by any means. They increase the risk of oesophageal and gastric perforation.

4 *The patient declines it.* The wish of a patient to refuse gastric lavage must be respected and to persist with it despite the patient's protestations is an offence in law. They can usually be persuaded to take an emetic.

Emesis or lavage?

The stomach can be emptied either by inducing vomiting or by passing a gastric lavage tube. It is doubtful if one is any more efficient than the other in recovering drugs and neither can be relied upon to empty the stomach completely. The method adopted will depend on the age, conscious level and degree of cooperation of the patient and the facilities and expertise available.

Gastric aspiration and lavage is appropriate for all unconscious patients and most adults who will cooperate. Induced emesis is the method of choice for children since a large enough tube cannot be passed and emesis is generally accepted as being psychologically less traumatic than passing a gastric tube. It should also be used in adults in whom gastric emptying is indicated but who refuse gastric lavage.

Induced emesis

Syrup of ipecacuanha is the most satisfactory agent for inducing emesis. Ipecacuanha Emetic Mixture, Paediatric (BP) is the formulation available in the UK. Recommended doses are 10 ml for children between the ages of 6 and 18 months, 15 ml for older children and 30 ml for adults. It is important that it is followed by a large drink (e.g. 200 ml of water for an adult). One dose will make about 70% of patients vomit within 20 minutes. If ineffective, the dose can be repeated after this time with success in a further 20%.

The use of salt and water to induce vomiting is unreliable and largely ineffective. In most cases it does no harm but in others, anxious relatives, eager to ensure rapid retrieval of the poison, may give grossly excessive quantities of salt and cause severe hypernatraemia. Several adults and children have died as a result and in many other deaths the role of salt may not have been appreciated. The use of saline emetics is therefore deprecated. Mechanical methods are inefficient and tartar emetic and copper sulphate solutions are potentially lethal.

Gastric aspiration and lavage
If indicated, gastric aspiration and lavage should be performed by the technique given in Appendix 3.

Complications and how to avoid them   *Oesophageal rupture* is a potentially fatal complication of gastric lavage but is extremely uncommon. It may be avoided by attention to the following:

1 Never carry out gastric lavage without good reason.
2 Lubricate the tube well with a suitable jelly.
3 Do not use force to pass the tube. Oesophageal perforation is most likely to occur when the patient is struggling. If the patient is uncooperative to this extent the need for gastric lavage should be reconsidered. Review the patient after an hour. If consciousness has been lost it may be possible to complete the procedure safely provided the airway can be safeguarded. On the other hand, if the patient's clinical state has not altered, it is doubtful if gastric emptying is indicated.
4 Do not attempt lavage in patients who have swallowed corrosive substances.

Following oesophageal perforation the patient may complain of central chest pain and rapidly becomes shocked with sweating, pallor, tachycardia and hypotension. Crepitus may be palpable in the root of the neck and subcutaneous and mediastinal emphysema may be seen on the chest X-ray. Fluids by mouth should be forbidden while an urgent contrast X-ray of the oesophagus or endoscopy is arranged to identify the point of rupture. Oesophagoscopy and closure of the perforation will be required and surgical advice should be sought immediately.

Inhalation of gastric contents is an ever-present hazard in unconscious and semiconscious patients. The risk may be reduced by observing the following:

1 Keep the patient on his or her left side in the semiprone or three-quarters prone position with the head slightly dependent during transport to hospital. Under no circumstance allow an unconscious patient to lie on his or her back.
2 Never give ipecac to patients who are likely to lose consciousness rapidly.
3 If the cough reflex is impaired, insert a cuffed endotracheal tube before attempting gastric lavage.
4 Always ensure that powerful suction apparatus (e.g. a Yankeur sucker) capable of removing large volumes of regurgitated fluid and particulate material is available and functioning before starting gastric lavage.

5 Take care to occlude the lumen of a lavage tube before withdrawing it because fluid remaining in the lumen may flood into the pharynx and be inhaled as the end of the tube emerges from the oesophagus.

The pulmonary response to inhalation of gastric content depends on several factors, including the volume inhaled, the pH of the fluid and the presence and size of food particles.

Experimental evidence indicates that the morbidity and mortality are particularly high when the pH of the aspirated fluid is less than 2.5. Acid fluid damages the lungs instantly and they rapidly become oedematous and haemorrhagic with areas of atelectasis due to reduced surfactant activity. Respiratory effort increases, bronchospasm may develop and arterial blood gas analysis usually shows a mixed respiratory and metabolic acidosis with hypoxaemia.

Inhalation of large food particles occasionally causes rapid death from laryngeal or tracheal obstruction whereas smaller particles cause lobar or segmental collapse. The role played by non-obstructing food particles in producing pulmonary damage is poorly understood but animal studies clearly demonstrate their ability to produce an extensive haemorrhagic pneumonia even when pH is neutral.

Treatment of laryngeal or major bronchus obstruction is a matter of the utmost urgency and laryngoscopy or bronchoscopy may be required to remove large food particles. However, bronchoscopy is hazardous in acutely hypoxic patients and is best avoided unless there is clear evidence of obstruction of a major airway. There is no evidence that bronchial lavage is helpful. In less severe cases it is usually sufficient to insert an endotracheal tube and carry out frequent bronchial suction which has the advantage of inducing coughing and thereby facilitates clearance of food fragments. It will not reduce the immediate pulmonary damage caused by acid and non-obstructing food particles. Frequent physiotherapy is essential.

Hypoxia may be corrected by increasing the inspired oxygen concentration but when severe, or associated with hypercapnia, assisted ventilation with or without positive end-expiratory pressure may be required. The most suitable method for individual cases is best decided in conjunction with anaesthetists.

It is traditional to give corticosteroids to patients who have inhaled gastric contents in the hope that pulmonary damage will be reduced, but there is no convincing evidence that they are beneficial.

Other supportive measures, including bronchodilators for bronchospasm and intravenous fluids for hypovolaemia, may be required. Antibiotics should be withheld until there is clear evidence of infection and an organism has been identified on Gram films or culture.

Lipoid pneumonia   The ingestion of petroleum distillate (long chain hydrocarbons) contained in paraffin, petrol, kerosene, turpentine substitute and furniture polishes may be complicated by aspiration into the lungs. The resulting acute inflammatory reaction in the alveoli and interstitial tissues is commonly referred to as a lipoid pneumonia. The hydrocarbon is phagocytosed by macrophages and can be identified in their cytoplasmic vacuoles.

The severity of symptoms caused by lipoid pneumonia is variable and there is no specific treatment. Antibiotics and corticosteroids have been recommended but the evidence for their efficacy is unconvincing. Whether the incidence of lipoid pneumonia can be minimized by not attempting to empty the stomach is controversial (p. 192).

Activated charcoal
It has been known for many years that charcoal can adsorb a large number of drugs and other toxins. Medicinal activated charcoal comprises granules of carbon formed by heating materials such as coconut shell, peat and wood in the absence of air until carbon is formed. The carbon is then 'activated' by exposing it to steam at high temperatures, as a consequence of which the number of internal channels within each particle and therefore the surface area available for adsorption of other substances is greatly increased. Manipulation of the manufacturing process can produce particles to required diameter and available surface area. Toxins which are adsorbed by charcoal are listed in Table 3.2 and those which are not in Table 3.3.

Table 3.2 Toxins which are adsorbed to activated charcoal

Barbiturates	Paracetamol
Benzodiazepines	Paraquat
Carbamazepine	Phenytoin
Chloroquine	Quinine
Dapsone	Salicylates
Digoxin	Theophylline
Digitoxin	

NB: Listing here does not necessarily imply therapeutic usefulness.

Table 3.3 Toxins which are not adsorbed to activated charcoal

Acids (strong)	Iron salts
Alkalis (strong)	Lithium salts
Cyanide salts	Methanol
Ethanol	Petroleum distillates
Ethylene glycol	

In some countries oral activated charcoal is widely used for the first-aid treatment of ingestion of potential toxins on the basis that administration within minutes will lead to the poison being adsorbed to the charcoal and not absorbed. With some drugs given to volunteers under fasting conditions, activated charcoal will reduce absorption by as much as 90%. However, if administration is delayed for an hour or more, the ability of activated charcoal to prevent absorption is greatly reduced. Activated charcoal may therefore be of value in the management of accidental poisoning in children but adults usually present too long after overdosage for it to be useful. However, such is the enthusiasm for activated charcoal that it is now being used in situations in which its value is not proven, it is unlikely to have any beneficial effect and morbidity and mortality are low in any case. Charcoal is not an easy option for patients or staff; patient acceptance is low and it is not entirely without adverse effects.

Formulations available   The available formulations of activated charcoal vary from one country to another. In the UK the choice lies between Medicoal and Carbomix. Both have to be mixed with water before use. The former is presented in 5 g sachets and is an effervescent preparation containing sodium citrate and povidone. Carbomix does not contain additives and comes in ready-to-use containers of 50 g to which the necessary volume of water can be added. The container is provided with an additional cap to facilitate administration down a nasogastric tube.

Limitations of use   The role of activated charcoal in the treatment of poisoning is limited by its acceptability to patients. It is a tasteless, black, gritty slurry which commonly causes vomiting, all of which tend to make patients decline to take it. Attempts to overcome these drawbacks by adding colouring and flavouring agents have had little success. The vomitus soils patients, staff and the surroundings, thereby straining relationships and generating additional work. More importantly, repeated doses of any charcoal have other adverse effects. With Medicoal, diarrhoea (which could be regarded as a therapeutic advantage) commonly develops while Carbomix and other charcoals which do not have additives tend to cause severe constipation and, rarely, the development of charcoal bezoars and even intestinal obstruction. The latter are sufficiently worrying to advise against overuse and giving a purgative when using charcoals which have no additives. Sorbitol is the one currently favoured, although it can cause hypernatraemia if given in excess. Any charcoal may be lethal if aspirated into the lungs.

Syrup of ipecac should not be given after activated charcoal since its emetine and alkaloid content will be adsorbed and rendered ineffective.

Dosage   Clearly, activated charcoal is not absorbed from the gut but is totally eliminated in the faeces. Systemic toxicity is therefore not a cause for concern, although local gut effects may limit use (see above). Consequently, dosage is not critical provided enough charcoal is given to adsorb the amount of poison ingested. However, about 10 times as much charcoal must be given as there is drug to be adsorbed and desirable doses usually have to be tempered in the interests of patient compliance. An acceptable guideline for the initial ('loading') dose is 1 g/kg body weight mixed with water to make a slurry.

Sorbitol is commercially available in 70% solutions. Only a single dose should be given. Adults should be given 50 ml of a 70% solution (diluted) and children 4.3 ml/kg of a 35% solution.

References

Allerton JP, Strom JA. Hypernatremia due to repeated oral doses of charcoal-sorbitol. *Am J Kidney Dis* 1991; **17**: 581–584.

Menzies DG, Busuttil A, Prescott LF. Fatal pulmonary aspiration of oral activated charcoal. *Br Med J* 1988; **297**: 459–460.

Pond SM. Role of repeated oral doses of activated charcoal in clinical toxicology. *Med Toxicol* 1986; **1**: 3–11.

Ray MJ, Padin DR, Condie JD *et al*. Charcoal bezoar. Small bowel obstruction secondary to amitriptyline overdose therapy. *Dig Dis Sci* 1988; **33**: 106–107.

Tenenbein M. Multiple doses of activated charcoal: time for reappraisal? *Ann Emerg Med* 1991; **20**: 529–531.

Whole-bowel irrigation

Whole-bowel irrigation is a method of evacuating the bowel contents rapidly and has been recommended for the treatment of poisoning with particularly toxic substances, sustained-release drug formulations (particularly when they have passed into the small bowel and are beyond recovery by gastric emptying) and with poisons which are not adsorbed by activated charcoal, especially iron. However, its value has not been adequately assessed.

The procedure usually involves passing a nasogastric tube, seating the patient on a commode and instilling the irrigation fluid into the stomach, although patients can occasionally be persuaded to drink the large volumes required. Watery diarrhoea soon develops and within 4–6 hours faecal material is usually absent from the rectal effluent. Initially, normal saline was used but it led to plasma volume expansion and hypokalaemia. Commercially available polyethylene glycol lavage solutions such as GoLytely and Klean-Prep (60 g/l polyethylene glycol together with electrolytes) are now recommended and are instilled at a rate of 2 l/hour in adults and 0.5 l/hour in preschool children. Limited observations suggest that patients tolerate whole-bowel irrigation well, even during pregnancy and infancy.

References

Everson GW, Bertaccini EJ, O'Leary J. Use of whole bowel irrigation in an infant following iron overdose. *Am J Emerg Med* 1991; **9**: 366–369.
Tenenbein M. Whole bowel irrigation as a gastrointestinal decontamination procedure after acute poisoning. *Med Toxicol* 1988; **3**: 77–84.
Van Ameyde KJ, Tenenbein M. Whole bowel irrigation during pregnancy. *Am J Obstet Gynecol* 1989; **160**: 646–647.

Body packing

Packets in the vagina can probably be removed digitally without risk of them rupturing but not those in the rectum.

The risks of swallowing packets are intestinal obstruction if they are made of strong material, or acute, usually massive, poisoning if they are fragile and rupture. The former is a clear indication for immediate surgery. The development of acute intoxication is also an indication for operative intervention, provided it is not so severe that it poses a risk for anaesthesia.

Not surprisingly, views on the management of patients who have not yet developed these complications are contradictory; some advocate surgery while others advise less invasive measures on the grounds that the incidence of complications is probably low. Induced emesis has successfully retrieved packets from the stomach and whole-bowel irrigation (p. 42) has induced rapid and safe elimination of those further down the gut. The toxicity and available treatment for poisoning with the drug involved are the critical factors in making decisions. Cannabis intoxication is unlikely to be lethal and naloxone is available to reverse opioid overdosage. A conservative attitude could therefore be justified with these drugs. In contrast, massive intoxication with cocaine, amphetamines and related substances is much less readily managed and carries a significant mortality. Early surgical intervention might be the best recommendation with these substances.

References

Hoffman RS, Smilkstein MJ, Goldfrank LR. Whole bowel irrigation and the cocaine body-packer. *Am J Emerg Med* 1990; **8**: 523–527.
Lancashire MJR, Legg PK, Lowe M *et al.* Surgical aspects of international drug smuggling. *Br Med J* 1988; **296**: 1035–1037.
Watson CJE, Thomson HJ, Johnston PS. Body-packing with amphetamines – an indication for surgery. *J R Soc Med* 1991; **84**: 311–312.

Emergency drug analysis

A venous blood sample should be taken for toxicological analysis from every patient admitted because of poisoning, the only exceptions being drug addicts or others who may be hepatitis B or human immunodeficiency virus (HIV) positive. In the latter cases blood should only be taken if mandatory for the management of the poisoning. As always, appropriate precautions must be taken to protect the person carrying out any procedure involving, and the laboratory staff handling, blood and other body fluids. If venesection is necessary in such patients a sample should be taken simultaneously for screening for Australia antigen.

There are two main reasons for taking blood for drug analysis:

1 In the important minority, to assess the severity of poisoning and the need for specific treatment.
2 For legal purposes should the patient die or develop some unexpected complication. It is therefore vital that the samples are accurately labelled with the patient's name, the date and time (24-hour clock) and kept refrigerated till the patient is discharged.

It will usually suffice to take 10 ml of blood into a lithium heparin tube. There are two exceptions to this rule: a plain tube must be used if it is intended to measure lithium concentrations, and blood for carboxyhaemoglobin estimations is best taken into heparinized syringes, taking care to exclude air. With lithium heparin samples it is preferable to separate the plasma and store it at <20°C if analysis is to be delayed.

In the vast majority of poisonings there is no justification for requesting an emergency drug analysis. Until recently it was common clinical practice to measure plasma concentrations of barbiturates routinely in unconscious patients but these investigations were done more to confirm the diagnosis and comfort the doctor than to alter management of the patient. Knowledge of the plasma barbiturate concentration is highly unlikely to make the clinician do anything more than continue to support vital functions. Salicylates rarely cause coma in adults and in the absence of other clinical features of salicylism, particularly hyperventilation, significant salicylate poisoning is unlikely. Requests for emergency drug analyses should be restricted to those poisonings where specific treatment is available and the need for it is determined from the plasma drug concentration. These include paracetamol, salicylate, iron, lithium, theophylline and possibly paraquat. Measurement of plasma drug concentrations is mandatory before attempting to enhance elimination by forced diuresis, haemodialysis or haemoperfusion. All unconscious poisoned patients should be screened for paracetamol since some have recovered from sedative overdoses only to become jaundiced and die from hepatic failure that might have been avoided had the early analysis of blood led to administration of specific treatment. Screening unconscious adults for paracetamol ingestion is far more important than looking for salicylates but, paradoxically, is much less commonly requested.

References

See p. 24.

Continuing care

Once emergency measures have been taken to maintain vital functions, the stomach has been emptied and antidotes, if available, have been administered, unconscious patients will require continuing intensive care. Their survival depends more on the standard of nursing care than on medical technology.

Respiratory care

General

Every unconscious patient should be nursed in the semiprone or three-quarters prone position unless an endotracheal tube has been inserted.

Secretions which collect in the oropharynx and especially in the dependent cheek should be removed regularly by suction. It is particularly important to do this before turning the patient from one side to the other to prevent aspiration of buccal secretions into the trachea. Removal of secretions in the mouth and pharynx is usually done blindly but if a rattle persists in the upper airway, direct laryngoscopy should be carried out to remove remaining secretions under direct vision.

Oropharyngeal tubes should be removed and inspected at 4-hour intervals and replaced if there is evidence that they are becoming blocked with secretions.

Intubated patients

If the patient has an endotracheal tube *in situ*, regular bronchial suction should be carried out using a sterile technique according to the amount of secretions to be removed. It is absolutely vital that the inspired air is adequately humidified and warmed to avoid drying and crusting of the tracheal mucosa and of secretions lying in the tube. The endotracheal tube should be removed once the patient starts to gag or have paroxysms of coughing and should be replaced by an oropharyngeal airway.

Daily samples of bronchial aspirate should be sent for bacteriological examination for as long as the patient is intubated. Antibiotics should not be given prophylactically to unconscious patients. A daily chest radiograph should be taken while the patient is unconscious or as indicated by the development of some respiratory complication.

Complications

Obstruction of endotracheal tubes. Endotracheal tubes may become obstructed in several ways including mechanical distortion, herniation of the inflated cuff over the end and by inspissation of secretions in the lumen. The latter can be prevented by carrying out regular bronchial suction and humidifying the inspired air while herniation of the cuff is highly unlikely if it is not overinflated. Kinking of the tube may be minimized by keeping the patient's neck slightly flexed.

Obstruction of the tube will cause a marked increase in inspiratory effort with indrawing of the intercostal spaces, soft tissues in the root of the neck and, in younger patients, the lower sternum. Central cyanosis will be present. Deflate the cuff and withdraw the tube immediately.

Aspiration pneumonia. Unconscious patients often aspirate pharyngeal secretions and are unable to clear them because the cough reflex is depressed. They are therefore likely to develop an aspiration pneumonia. This complication is usually suspected from the findings on clinical examination of the lungs, fever or purulent bronchial secretions and is confirmed by chest radiography. A Gram film of bronchial aspirate should be made and appropriate antibiotic therapy begun before the results of culture are available. If no organism is obvious on the direct film a broad-spectrum antibiotic such as amoxycillin should be given and changed later if necessary. Frequent bronchial suction and intensive physiotherapy are mandatory. Bronchoscopy should be reserved for patients with lobar collapse.

If respiratory infection is severe and life-threatening, consider methods of shortening the duration of coma in order to speed the return of an effective cough reflex.

Skin care

Unconscious patients should be turned from one side to the other at 2-hour intervals or more frequently if skin lesions are present. Careful attention must be given to skin over bony prominences to avoid pressure sores.

Bullous lesions should be kept intact for as long as possible to reduce the likelihood of infection, but once they burst, the roof should be removed and the denuded area covered with a sterile, absorbent, non-stick dressing until exudation stops. The dressing should be replaced daily or more frequently, depending on the amount of discharge. When the discharge stops or is minimal the area should be left exposed to dry and crust over.

Eye care

Blinking is abolished in unconscious patients and great care must be taken to ensure that the eyelids are kept closed, taping them down if necessary, to avoid exposure keratitis. Instillation of methylcellulose eye drops into the conjunctival sac, three or four times daily, will also be helpful.

Some patients who are kept lying horizontally without pillows, or who have been nursed in a head-down position because of hypotension, rapidly develop marked subconjunctival, eyelid and facial oedema. This may be the result of posture but a drug effect on blood vessels may also contribute. It is of little importance in itself but may reflect a tendency to oedema in the upper respiratory tract and, if the blood pressure permits, the head should be raised above body level, preferably by tilting the whole bed.

Fluid balance

Many patients (e.g. those poisoned with benzodiazepines and tricyclic antidepressants) do not require intravenous fluids since most are able to drink within 12–24 hours. However, in severely poisoned patients a venous line should be inserted in case urgent drug therapy is necessary. The temptation to give large volumes of intravenous fluids must be resisted. Barbiturates, opioid analgesics and other CNS depressants have antidiuretic effects and unconscious, hypoventilating and hypothermic patients have reduced insensible fluid losses. It is therefore unnecessary to give more than 2 l of fluid intravenously in 24 hours. Nor is there any need to start until the patient has been unconscious for 24 hours. When maintenance fluids are indicated 5% dextrose (1.0 l) and 0.9% saline (0.5 l) in rotation are usually adequate but should be altered as indicated by the plasma electrolytes.

Bladder care

The bladder in most unconscious patients can usually be emptied by applying firm suprapubic pressure. The great majority of poisoned adults admitted in coma will be conscious within 12 hours, will produce relatively little urine during that time and will not be grateful to find themselves catheterized unnecessarily. The indications for catheterization are given on p. 53.

Hypothermia

Simple measures
Hypothermia is seldom severe and the rectal temperature rarely falls below 30°C. Usually only simple measures are required for its

correction and there is no virtue in attempting rapid correction in acute poisoning. The patient should be nursed in a normally warm room and covered with a reasonable number of blankets. It is customary to wrap the patient in a sheet of aluminiumized plastic to reflect back radiant heat from the body but this type of covering is no more efficient than ordinary plastic sheeting. The latter is therefore useful in the first-aid situation. The efficiency of both materials is reduced if moisture condenses on the inner aspect of the sheet and this can be minimized by placing a blanket between the patient and the plastic cover. It is important that hypothermic patients are unwrapped for as short periods as possible and to the least extent for nursing and medical procedures. These measures will usually produce a slow return of body temperature to normal.

Other measures
Various more elaborate techniques have been used to correct hypothermia. These include heating one forearm in a water bath at 37°C or using a soda lime canister as a heat exchanger to warm inspired air. In extreme cases haemodialysis or irrigation of the mediastinum or peritoneal cavity with warm fluids has been used but it is very doubtful if such heroic measures can ever be justified for the treatment of hypothermia alone. Body temperature usually rises as the level of consciousness improves and patients whose hypothermia is refractory to simple treatment are likely to be severely poisoned or elderly. Procedures to enhance elimination of the poison may be indicated.

Increasing elimination of poisons

General considerations

Various techniques have been used in attempts to enhance the elimination of poisons, including exchange transfusion, forced diuresis, peritoneal dialysis, haemodialysis, haemoperfusion through charcoal and ion exchange resins, and plasmapheresis. Unfortunately, the enthusiasm with which they have been advocated has not always been founded on critical appraisal of their efficacy and their role in the management of acute poisoning is now extremely limited, partly because the toxins for which they were useful have become much less common with the changing pattern of drug prescribing (at least in developed countries) and partly because of the realization that repeated doses of oral activated charcoal ('gut dialysis') can be almost as effective.

Forced diuresis, in particular, has been used excessively and inappropriately, occasionally with fatal consequences and there is an increasing body of opinion that it now has no role. Exchange transfusion is an inefficient method of eliminating poisons and even in childhood has very little place as a therapeutic manoeuvre. The role of plasmapheresis has yet to be defined.

When active elimination of a poison is indicated the choice usually lies between repeated oral charcoal, haemodialysis or charcoal haemoperfusion. Peritoneal dialysis has only about 20% the efficiency of haemodialysis but may still be useful in the initial management of severe poisoning with toxins which can be removed by haemodialysis pending transfer of the patient to a centre able to carry out haemodialysis. Clearly elimination techniques are not indicated in poisoning with compounds for which there is a specific antidote or with those such as benzodiazepines which are relatively harmless in overdosage.

Repeat-dose oral activated charcoal

Administration of oral activated charcoal at 2- or 4-hourly intervals for the duration of toxicity has now become one of the most important and widely applicable methods of enhancing elimination of toxins from the circulation. Its use results from the observation that repeated oral doses of charcoal greatly shortened the plasma half-life of phenobarbitone given intravenously to volunteers. Although some of this effect may be due to interruption of enterohepatic circulation of drugs (e.g. phenobarbitone and cardiac glycosides), it is more probable that by maintaining virtually zero drug concentrations in the gut lumen, the charcoal causes a gradient, by means of which drug can move from plasma in the capillaries of the intestinal villi to the lumen where it is bound. The process has therefore attracted the designation 'gut dialysis'. The substances for which the technique is most helpful are listed in Table 3.2 (p. 40). Metallic ions are not adsorbed and of the drugs, those with an acidic nature are best adsorbed.

Dosage and adverse effects

Charcoal dosage, the need for concomitant purgative administration and the adverse effects of repeated doses are discussed on p. 41. The first dose should be a loading dose and the full amount or half-dose should be repeated at 4- or 2-hour intervals respectively until signs of toxicity clear or the patient will not tolerate further amounts.

Haemodialysis

Haemodialysis is an effective method of increasing the elimination of small molecules (molecular weight <350 Da) which cross semipermeable membranes readily. Maximum removal of poison depends on the following factors:

1 The plasma concentration of the poison should be high to produce a steep diffusion gradient between plasma and dialyser bath fluid. The common poisons most likely to satisfy this criterion are salicylates, phenobarbitone, ethylene glycol, methanol, lithium and potassium.
2 Protein and tissue binding of the poison should be as small as possible because the diffusion gradient depends on the plasma concentration of free drug rather than on the total drug concentration.
3 The poison should be water-soluble rather than lipid-soluble. This criterion to some extent explains the success of haemodialysis in removing salicylates and phenobarbitone.
4 The volume of distribution of the poison should be as small as possible. Compounds such as lithium and potassium are readily dialysable and plasma concentrations can be reduced rapidly by haemodialysis. Unfortunately their volume of distribution is large so that plasma concentrations quickly rebound within a few hours of stopping dialysis. It is therefore preferable to use an alternative treatment.

Most of the serious poisonings encountered in clinical practice are unsuitable for treatment by haemodialysis. Tricyclic antidepressants have a large volume of distribution with plasma concentrations too low for haemodialysis to be of value. Haemodialysis still has a role in severe salicylate poisoning and possibly in phenobarbitone poisoning, though haemoperfusion is more efficient in the latter.

Haemoperfusion

The ability of activated charcoal to adsorb drugs has been known for many years. It is given orally to reduce the absorption of ingested poisons and was used in the filters of gas masks in the last World War to adsorb various gases. In 1962 a Greek physician published an account of the use of activated charcoal to remove drugs from the blood of poisoned adults.

Technical considerations
The technique is simple. Arterial blood is led from the radial artery to the bottom of a cylinder packed with granules of activated charcoal and primed with saline. The blood is allowed to percolate through the charcoal and is filtered at the top of the cylinder and returned to the patient through a convenient vein. This technique has now been shown to remove a wide variety of drugs, particularly the barbiturate hypnotics

and glutethimide which are poorly dialysable, and has the advantages of being more efficient and simpler to use than haemodialysis. Initially, however, it was not without some disadvantages. Hypotension, charcoal embolization, leucopenia and, more seriously, thrombocytopenia were common. Fragmentation and embolization of charcoal particles has now been eliminated by coating the granules with an acrylic hydrogel at the expense of only a slight reduction in adsorbing capacity. The platelet count falls by 25–50% in the first 2 hours of haemoperfusion but then rises despite continuation of the procedure. Haemorrhagic complications occasionally arise but are uncommon.

Clinical use
The advent of charcoal haemoperfusion was a major advance in the treatment of severe poisoning with CNS depressant drugs including barbiturate hypnotics, phenobarbitone, glutethimide, methaqualone, ethchlorvynol and meprobamate, but these drugs are now largely obsolete and overdosage with them has almost disappeared. Unfortunately, the evidence suggests that this technique does not remove significant quantities of tricyclic antidepressants which are amongst the most toxic CNS depressants encountered today. Haemoperfusion will therefore only be required by a small minority of very severely poisoned patients and it should be regarded as an adjunct to, rather than a substitute for, meticulous supportive care. Patients suitable for charcoal haemoperfusion should satisfy the first and at least one other of the following criteria:

1 The plasma concentration should not be less than:

Drug	Concentration (mg/l)
Barbiturate hypnotics	50
Ethchlorvynol	150
Glutethimide	50
Meprobamate	100
Methaqualone	40
Phenobarbitone	150
Theophylline	100

2 Poisoning must be clinically severe, with grade 4 coma, hypothermia, hypotension and respiratory depression.
3 The patient's clinical state should be deteriorating or failing to improve despite supportive care.

4 Serious complications should be present, e.g. hepatic and renal insufficiency or extensive pneumonia while the patient is still unconscious.

References

Pond SM. Extracorporeal techniques in the treatment of poisoned patients. *Med J Aust* 1991; **154**: 617–622.

Winchester JF. Poisoning: is the role of the nephrologist diminishing? *Am J Kidney Dis* 1989; **13**: 171–183.

Complications of poisoning

Complications occurring during the course of acute poisoning may be due to predictable, but uncommon, effects of the poison or to chance events resulting from impaired consciousness.

Pulmonary oedema

Pulmonary oedema complicating poisoning may be cardiac or non-cardiac in aetiology. The former is far more common and is usually the result of gross fluid overload during forced diuresis. In many cases there is no pharmacokinetic justification for attempting forced diuresis; in others no allowance is made for the possible nephrotoxic or myocardial depressant effects of the poison itself. The antidiuretic effect of some drugs (e.g. opioid analgesics, barbiturates, salicylates and paracetamol) may also be an important aetiological factor. Fatalities occur and are all the more tragic since most are avoidable. This variety of pulmonary oedema should be treated conventionally by stopping fluid administration and giving diuretics and oxygen. If renal failure is present, dialysis may be necessary to remove the excess fluid.

Non-cardiac pulmonary oedema occurs with some inhaled toxins (ammonia, chlorine, oxides of nitrogen) and with ingestion of salicylates, opioid analgesics, paraquat, ethchlorvynol. This form of pulmonary oedema does not respond to diuretics and digoxin but may to corticosteroids which should be given in full doses.

Renal failure

Acute renal failure due to renal tubular necrosis is a relatively uncommon complication of acute poisoning and is usually the result of a combination of factors, including hypotension, hypoxia and a predictable direct effect of the poison on tubular cells (e.g. paraquat, salicylate, paracetamol, carbon tetrachloride). Rarely gross intravascular haemolysis or myoglobinuria may be the cause. Even in the absence of these factors, some drugs (e.g. heroin) cause marked, unexplained reduction in effective renal plasma flow and glomerular filtration rate.

Renal failure may be anticipated from the patient's history and condition and strongly suspected when oliguria (urine volume <500 ml/ 24 hours) develops. Urinary retention should always be excluded as a possible cause of apparent oliguria. Urine production should be recorded carefully and 24-hour collections kept for measurement of osmolality and electrolytes. Conscious patients are usually able to void naturally if a large enough volume is present in the bladder. Indiscriminate catheterization of all unconscious patients cannot be justified and should be reserved for:

1 Patients with retention that cannot be relieved by suprapubic pressure.
2 Those in coma who are undergoing forced diuresis.
3 When there is a strong suspicion of renal failure.

The plasma urea and electrolytes should be measured daily. If there is a likelihood of concurrent hepatocellular damage the plasma creatinine should also be measured since it is a more reliable indicator of renal failure than the urea under these circumstances. The central venous pressure should be assessed by insertion of a central venous line and the intravascular volume expanded with plasma as necessary. It may then be possible to initiate a diuresis by giving adults frusemide (0.25 or 0.5 g intravenously over 20 min). Careful fluid balance throughout is mandatory and intake should be adjusted to the urine volume in the preceding 24 hours with an additional 0.5 l to make up for insensible loss. Most acutely poisoned patients with renal failure are too ill to want to eat and dietary protein restriction is irrelevant. If, despite these measures, the plasma urea or creatinine continues to rise, the patient's blood should be screened for hepatitis B surface antigen and the patient referred for haemofiltration or haemodialysis.

Cerebral oedema

Generalized cerebral oedema is frequently found in fatal cases of acute poisoning (particularly in liver failure secondary to paracetamol overdosage) and may well be present in others who are desperately ill but survive. It is produced by various factors operating simultaneously, including hypoxia and hypercapnia due to respiratory failure, hypotension (the effects of which may have been potentiated by posture), hypoglycaemia and possibly drug-induced impairment of capillary integrity. The majority of patients who develop cerebral oedema probably do so before admission to hospital, though in others it may be the consequence of refractory hypotension or protracted cardio-respiratory resuscitation. Diagnosis is usually a matter of conjecture but a computed tomography scan may help. Treatment includes correction of hypoxia, hypercapnia and hypotension but in severely poisoned patients the latter may be extremely difficult until attempts are made to enhance the elimination of the poison. Hyperventilation of the patient till the $Paco_2$ lies between 3.0 and 3.4 kPa (22 and 25 mmHg) has been recommended for some forms of cerebral oedema but its feasibility and value in poisoned patients may be offset by coexisting severe hypotension. Mannitol 1 g/kg body weight in the form of a 20% solution should be given intravenously. Dexamethasone intramuscularly is recommended for longer-term management but it is not always effective in patients with generalized brain oedema. The patient should be nursed with the head elevated and fluid administration should be kept to the minimum.

Convulsions

Convulsions may complicate poisoning with many drugs, including CNS stimulants, anticholinergic compounds and non-steroidal anti-inflammatory agents. If they are isolated and of brief duration, treatment is unnecessary but if frequently recurring or protracted they should be treated with intravenous diazepam. Patients who have a combination of vomiting and convulsions are at particular risk of inhalation of gastric contents and it may be safer to paralyse and ventilate them mechanically until the poison has been metabolized and excreted. If this approach is adopted, monitor cerebral function and suppress seizure activity with anticonvulsants.

Rhabdomyolysis and peripheral nerve injuries

Patients who lie unconscious in the same posture for long periods are in danger of muscle and nerve injuries.

Muscles subjected to protracted pressure frequently become necrotic and this may account for the elevation of serum enzyme levels known to occur in unconscious poisoned patients. Some poisons which have been associated are listed in Table 3.4. Convulsions may contribute to the muscle damage and there is often associated hyperthermia. Myoglobinuria may also result and contribute to the development of renal failure. Myositis ossificans has been reported as a long-term complication, particularly after poisoning with barbiturates and carbon monoxide, but is an extremely rare sequel. Rarely, rhabdomyolysis may cause such an increase in muscle compartment pressure (particularly in

Table 3.4 Toxins which have been associated with rhabdomyolysis

Amoxapine	Isopropanol	Phencyclidine
Barbiturates	Methadone	Phenelzine
Caffeine	Methyl ethyl ketone peroxide	Protriptyline
Carbon monoxide	Nitrazepam	Pseudoephedrine
Cocaine	Opioid analgesics	Salicylates
Diphenhydramine	Oxprenolol	Strychnine
Doxepin	Paracetamol	Terbutaline
Doxylamine	Paraphenylene diamine	Theophylline
Heroin	Pemoline	Toluene
Isoniazid	Pentaborane	

the lower leg) that the arterial blood supply to the distal limb is severely impaired and emergency fasciotomy is required.

Some peripheral nerves are at particular risk of direct compression damage. They are the radial, ulnar and lateral peroneal which lie relatively superficially and in relationship to bone. The damage is not usually evident until the patient regains consciousness and complains of numbness, paraesthesiae or weakness in the distribution of the nerve involved. Recovery is usually complete but may take several weeks or months.

These nerves may also be damaged indirectly by extensive oedema and swelling within fascial compartments or be caught up in fibrous tissue as necrotic skeletal muscle heals.

References

Curry SC, Chang D, Connor D. Drug- and toxin-induced rhabdomyolysis. *Ann Emerg Med* 1989; **18**: 1068–1084.

Köppel C. Clinical features, pathogenesis and management of drug-induced rhabdomyolysis. *Med Toxicol* 1989; **4**: 108–126.

Taniguchi Y, Wada D, Takahashi M *et al*. Multiple bullae and paresis after drug-induced coma. *Acta Dermatol Venereol* 1991; **18**: 536–538.

Postextubation laryngeal oedema

Some degree of laryngeal oedema probably occurs in every patient who has been intubated for more than a few hours but it seldom causes symptoms. In occasional cases, however, rebound hyperaemia of the cords with rapid accumulation of oedema may cause life-threatening laryngeal obstruction after extubation. It is particularly likely to develop in young women in whom the larynx tends to be relatively small and in whom the diameter of the endotracheal tube that can be accommodated is critical. Fluid overload and lying in a head-down posture are also important aetiological factors.

Laryngeal oedema should be suspected when the patient develops stridor and signs of major airway obstruction within a few hours of extubation. Most settle when propped up to allow gravity to help reduce oedema and after being given warm, humidified, oxygen-enriched air by face mask. In severe cases tracheostomy may be necessary but should be avoided if at all possible, particularly in young women who will have to carry a prominent scar as a constant reminder of the episode for the rest of their lives.

Rare complications

Rare complications of acute poisoning include acute gastric dilatation and paralytic ileus. Respiratory tract burns may occur as a result of inhalation of hot, stimulant beverages administered to drowsy patients in well-intentioned, but futile, attempts to prevent them losing consciousness. Spinal artery thrombosis with consequent paraplegia rarely complicates prolonged, severe, hypotension.

The recovery period and after-care

Recovery

Disturbed behaviour

During recovery from overdoses of psychotropic drugs patients may exhibit grossly disturbed behaviour and can be a danger to themselves and others. This is commonly seen in association with tricyclic antidepressants and other anticholinergic compounds when patients frequently become agitated, delirious and hallucinate for 2 or 3 days. Large doses of diazepam may be required (p. 69).

Behaviour disturbance during recovery from barbiturate poisoning differs, particularly with phenobarbitone. The patient is usually disinhibited, loquacious, dysarthric, readily amused or, in some cases, aggressive and resentful of attention. In an unsupervised moment they may try to climb out of bed, often in a state of undress, and injure themselves. For their safety, to reduce subsequent embarrassment and for the peace of mind of relatives and staff, sedation is necessary. One dose of chlorpromazine (25–50 mg intramuscularly for an adult) is usually sufficient but some require more. This disinhibited state may be particularly prolonged and troublesome when phenobarbitone has been taken and in addition to sedation, repeated oral charcoal may be indicated.

Psychiatric and social assessment

Following recovery from the physical effects of self-poisoning the patient should be interviewed to determine the cause for the episode and to identify any psychiatric illness or social precipitant which can be corrected. Whether this should be done by psychiatrists and social workers or by suitably trained general physicians is a matter of debate and will depend on the attitudes and enthusiasm of all concerned and the local availability of social and psychiatric services at short notice. Regardless of who accepts the role, it is essential that assessment is carried out as soon as possible after the overdose. Giving the patient an appointment to attend a psychiatric outpatient clinic at some time in the future is totally unsatisfactory because the default rate is so high.

Unfortunately, despite intensive psychiatric and social assessment, about 15–20% of patients return within a year with another episode of self-poisoning, most occurring within 3 months of the first. The reasons are not difficult to identify:

1 Little can be done to reduce disagreement and violence between sexual partners and the reconciliation resulting from the first episode is often fragile and breaks down with little provocation. Advice to the partners to separate is often unrealistic since, in present-day society, tenancy of the home is usually in the man's name and the woman may have no refuge to which she can go.
2 Treatment for alcoholism, drug dependence and personality disorders is not nearly as successful as one would wish.
3 Psychiatric illness tends to relapse unpredictably.
4 The inherent nature of some of these individuals is such that they may create more of life's minor crises than the population as a whole and they are often less able to cope with them.
5 Involvement in crime is high among men who repeat self-poisoning and is not readily reduced.
6 Problems of substandard housing, high-rise living and unemployment require political rather than medical solutions.
7 The real patient may not be the individual who has taken the overdose but perhaps the violent, alcoholic husband who does not know, or will not accept, that he has a problem.

The clinician may not only predict and be unable to prevent the dissolution of many partnerships but, even more seriously, the inevitability of episodes of self-poisoning in any offspring. Self-poisoning in teenagers is frequently associated with conflict with parents, truancy, failure to attain academic performance compatible with intelligence, early experimentation with drugs and alcohol and involvement in petty crime. These are the most depressing and disturbing facets of self-poisoning but when one considers the incidence of precipitating factors in the population it becomes surprising that the repeat rate is so low. Many people must come to terms with what others would consider to be appalling circumstances and they deserve sympathy, under-standing and help. Government at all levels must also help find solutions to some of the problems.

Review of regular drug treatment

General considerations

Following recovery from an episode of self-poisoning, the opportunity should be taken to review the patient's regular drug treatment. Despite their low average age, many are on regular treatment, particularly with psychotropic drugs which they may have been taking for weeks, months or even years. It is commonplace to meet patients who have been taking two or three different types of psychotropic drug concurrently (e.g. a tranquillizer, antidepressant and hypnotic). It must also be remembered that about 60% of patients who take drug overdoses do so with medicines which they have been prescribed and another 15% take drugs which have been prescribed for close relatives. Rationalization of prescribing may help reduce morbidity related to regular drug ingestion and also diminish the availability of drugs for repeated episodes of self-poisoning.

Benzodiazepines

Benzodiazepines comprise the single most important group of drugs given to those who present with self-poisoning, usually young and middle-aged women who are unduly anxious, have marital problems, difficulty in coping with children and a variety of other social stresses. Clearly drugs cannot resolve these problems but they may blunt the individual's response to them and make them more tolerable. On the other hand, it is possible that some patients become so drugged that they are even less capable of coping than they were in the first place. When questioned, some patients spontaneously admit that tranquillizers were unhelpful or made them even more depressed. It has also been suggested that benzodiazepines, like alcohol, release aggression and fuel the interpersonal conflict which so commonly precedes self-poisoning. Commonly, one meets patients who have been prescribed two and occasionally three different benzodiazepines, presumably in the mistaken belief that their actions are radically different. Psychiatric patients in particular are likely to get into difficulties if drugs are prescribed by the hospital and by the family doctor concurrently. Fortunately, the level of prescribing of benzodiazepines shows some signs of falling as all concerned become aware of the problems of dependence and doctors, whether by education or fear of litigation resulting from dependence, are less liberal with pills which have no hope of changing social stresses. However, many patients continue to demand them.

Analgesics
Analgesics are another group of drugs which may be prescribed for long periods and have effects on cerebral function. This is particularly true of the opioid analgesics, dextropropoxyphene, dihydrocodeine and dipipanone, especially if prescribed in conjunction with tranquillizers, antidepressants, hypnotics or anticonvulsants.

On other occasions patients may be taking drugs with contrary actions on the CNS (e.g. appetite suppressants which stimulate the brain and benzodiazepines or hypnotics which depress it, ergotamine preparations for migraine and vasodilators because of cold hands, phenothiazines and anticholinergic drugs, depressants and antidepressants). There is considerable scope for the rationalization of drug treatment or even the discontinuation of some drugs in most patients.

Advice about driving

Recovery from minor overdoses of psychotropic drugs appears to take place very quickly and the patient is soon able to walk steadily, talk coherently and to be interviewed. This may lull the physician into thinking that the effects of the drugs have disappeared completely · before the patient is discharged. However, this is not the case and many drugs, most importantly the benzodiazepines, have persistent active metabolites, which will continue to act on the brain for several days or weeks after the overdose. These may be sufficient to impair coordination and reflexes and therefore the ability to perform complex tasks such as driving a motor vehicle or operating complicated machinery with safety. The doctor clearly has a responsibility to the general public as well as to the individual recovering from the drug overdose. The patient must be warned against participating in such activities for a variable period of time, the length of which has to be judged from a knowledge of the drugs involved in individual cases. It must also be stressed to the patient that the effects of alcohol will be potentiated during this time.

Points of emphasis

- All but a small minority of unconscious poisoned patients recover with supportive care alone.
- A clear airway is imperative.
- Improving the airway alone may improve ventilation, hypotension and level of consciousness.
- Arterial blood gas analysis is essential for the assessment of ventilation.

- Arterial hydrogen ion concentrations and oxygen and carbon dioxide tensions should no longer be corrected for body temperature.
- Hypotension usually responds to simple measures to increase venous return.
- Correct hypercapnia before correcting metabolic acidosis.
- Consult the poisons information services if you are in doubt about the constituents, toxicity or treatment of poisoning with any product.
- Speak personally to a physician at the poisons information service if there is difficulty.
- Antidotes, particularly for opioid analgesics, paracetamol and iron salts, may be life-saving.
- Induced emesis using syrup of ipecacuanha is the method of choice for emptying the stomach in conscious children.
- Never use salt solution as an emetic.
- Never attempt gastric emptying by any method if the airway cannot be protected.
- Emergency drug analyses are only indicated if the result will alter management.
- Measurement of plasma drug concentrations is mandatory before attempting forced diuresis, haemodialysis and haemoperfusion to eliminate drugs.
- Humidify and warm the air for patients with endotracheal tubes.
- Manage skin blisters as burns.
- The eyes of unconscious patients must be kept lubricated and closed to avoid exposure damage.
- Unconscious poisoned patients seldom require more than 2.0 litres of intravenous fluid daily.
- Indiscriminate catheterization of every unconscious patient is unacceptable.
- Hypothermia does not require rapid correction or heroic treatment.
- Charcoal haemoperfusion should be used to eliminate CNS depressants – but only in very severe poisoning.
- Pulmonary oedema complicating acute poisoning is often the result of misguided attempts to force a diuresis.
- Renal failure should be treated conventionally.
- Cerebral oedema should be anticipated in patients who have had prolonged hypotension or cardiorespiratory arrest.
- Disturbed behaviour is common during recovery.
- Every patient who has deliberately poisoned him- or herself must be assessed to identify correctable psychiatric and social precipitants.
- Review the patient's drug treatment after self-poisoning.
- Advise the patient about driving and other complex tasks after overdosage with psychotropic drugs.

Chapter 4

Features and management of specific poisons

Acetone

General considerations

Acetone is a volatile and inflammable organic solvent widely used in laboratories and domestically for nail varnish removal. It is one of the solvents abused by 'glue sniffers' and can be absorbed through the lungs, skin and alimentary tract. Childhood exposures are common but serious poisoning is rare. The plasma half-life of acetone varies from 13 to 30 hours.

Features

Depression of consciousness and respiration and convulsions are the most serious consequences. The breath smells of acetone and the throat may be inflamed, oedematous and show superficial ulceration if the acetone has been ingested. Hyperglycaemia (usually not more than 200 mg/dl or 11 mmol/l) and glycosuria have been reported and the oral glucose tolerance curve may be diabetic in character. The mechanism of glucose intolerance is not known. Acetone will be present in the urine. Liver function is not disturbed.

Management

The patient should be removed from the toxic atmosphere and contaminated clothing must be removed and the skin thoroughly washed. There is probably little merit in emptying the stomach if only a small amount of acetone has been ingested and to do so after large quantities is contraindicated because of the corrosive actions of the chemical. Supportive measures will be required if the patient is unconscious but there is no specific treatment. Treatment for hyperglycaemia will not usually be required.

Prognosis

Recovery of consciousness may be anticipated within a few hours. Glucose tolerance may take a few months to return to normal.

Reference

Gamis AS, Wasserman GS. Acute acetone intoxication in a pediatric patient. *Pediatr Emerg Care* 1988; 4: 24–26.

Adder envenomation

General considerations

The adder, *Vipera berus*, is found widely throughout Western Europe and is the only naturally occurring poisonous snake in the UK. Bites usually result from trying to pick up the snake but may also occur if it is taken unawares. They are only likely to be encountered in the summer months since the adder hibernates during the winter. Probably less than 50% of bites are associated with the injection of venom.

Features

The bite comprises two puncture marks about a centimetre apart and usually occurs on the extremity of a limb. It may go unnoticed until swelling develops but more often there is immediate pain. Swelling at the site is usually apparent within an hour and is a certain indicator of the injection of venom. However, systemic poisoning may occur in the absence of local reaction. Vomiting, abdominal pain and diarrhoea may occur within a few minutes and occasionally transient hypotension and loss of consciousness also occur at a very early stage. Gastrointestinal symptoms may continue for 2 days and over this time the limb swelling extends and becomes haemorrhagic, blood loss often being sufficient to cause anaemia after a few days. In the worst cases the trunk, face and lips may become swollen. Hypotension may persist or occur up to 36 hours after the bite and this, together with development of bleeding, oliguria, a neutrophil leucocytosis and non-specific electrocardiogram changes indicates severe systemic poisoning.

Management

First aid
Reassurance of the victim is one of the most important aspects of first aid. The bite should not be incised or sucked but cleaned and covered with a dry dressing. If hospital is more than 30 minutes away a bandage

or light ligature should be placed round the limb proximal to the bite and should be tight enough to impede venous return without obstructing arterial inflow. If practicable the limb should not be used since muscle activity will facilitate absorption of venom from the bite. The affected limb should be kept dependent.

Hospital referral
Every victim should be referred to hospital and observed for at least 24 hours.

General measures
Remove any ligature that is present. Symptomatic treatment may be required for undue anxiety, pain or vomiting but antibiotics, corticosteroids and antitetanus treatment are unnecessary. Local application of ice-packs may add to tissue necrosis and should not be used.

Investigation and monitoring
The pulse rate and blood pressure should be recorded hourly for 48 hours and a careful note made of the urinary output and the volumes of fluid lost through vomiting and diarrhoea. Assess and record the extent of swelling daily (or more frequently in the first day or two of envenomation) by measuring the girth of the proximal and distal parts of the affected and contralateral limbs about the midpoints.

The white cell count, plasma urea and electrolytes should be measured daily. An electrocardiogram should be performed twice dally or the cardiac rhythm monitored continuously if hypotension is present. A coagulation screen is indicated if bleeding occurs.

Antivenom
The only antivenom which is generally available and of value is the Zagreb antivenom. Clinical trials of a viper-specific Fab-fragment antibody have just commenced.

Indications   The principal indications for the use of Zagreb antivenom are:

1 Persistent or recurrent hypotension.
2 Bleeding.
3 Electrocardiogram changes.
4 Leucocytosis ($20\,000/mm^3$ or greater).
5 In adults in whom swelling has extended up the limb within 2 hours of the bite, to reduce disability from the local effects of the poison.

Contraindications   The benefits of antivenom have to be weighed against the risk of hypersensitivity reactions to the serum, and a history of asthma or other allergic condition is therefore a relative contra-indication to its use. However, recent evidence suggests that it is remarkably safe. The subcutaneous injection of a small dose as a test of serum hypersensitivity is of no value and may give misleading results.

Administration
1 0.5 ml of 1:1000 adrenaline (0.5 mg) *must* be drawn into a syringe *before* giving antivenom.
2 Two ampoules (a total of 4 ml) of European viper venom antiserum (Institute of Immunology, Zagreb) should be added to 100 ml normal saline and infused at a rate of 15 drops/minute. Note that the dose does not vary with age.
3 Immediate reactions to antivenom can be satisfactorily controlled by temporarily stopping the infusion and prompt intramuscular injection of the adrenaline.

Prognosis

Death from adder envenomation is extremely rare and many more deaths have been reported from bee and wasp stings. Patients under the age of 14 years usually recover completely in 3 weeks or less while many adults take significantly longer.

References

Cederholm I, Lennmarken C. *Vipera berus* bites in children – experience of early antivenom treatment. *Acta Paediatr Scand* 1987; **76**: 682–684.
Hawley A. Adder bites in Aldershot. *J R Army Med Corps* 1988; **134**: 135–137.
Moore RS. Second-degree heart block associated with envenomation by *Vipera berus*. *Arch Emerg Med* 1988; **5**: 116–118.

Alpha-chloralose

General considerations

Alpha-chloralose is used as an animal anaesthetic and to kill rodents, bird pests and moles. The rodenticide preparations comprise cereal baits containing 4% alpha-chloralose while technical alpha-chloralose (about 90% pure) is used against moles and is occasionally encountered in self-poisoning episodes. The toxic amount for an adult is said to be 1 g and for an infant, 20 mg/kg body weight.

Features

Ingestion of prepared rodenticide baits is unlikely to cause toxicity unless a very large quantity is eaten. Despite being used as an anaesthetic, the toxic effects of alpha-chloralose are those of severe central nervous system (CNS) excitation and are similar to those of intoxication with strychnine. Hypersalivation, increased muscle tone, hyperreflexia, opisthotonus and convulsions are the major effects and rhabdomyolysis is a potential complication. Coma, generalized flaccidity and respiratory depression may follow.

Management

No treatment is required for most children who ingest alpha-chloralose baits. Supportive measures are necessary when very large amounts of bait or the technical compound is involved. A clear airway and adequate ventilation must be maintained. Convulsions should be suppressed with intravenous diazepam but if control cannot be attained with acceptable quantities (no more than 30 mg in an adult), it may be necessary to paralyse and ventilate the patient while monitoring cerebral function and suppressing seizure activity with larger doses or with another drug. Repeated doses of oral activated charcoal should be given when control of the airway and convulsions has been achieved but gastric emptying is best not carried out to avoid unnecessary stimulation of the patient which might provoke further seizures.

Reference

Thomas HM, Simpson D, Prescott LF. The toxic effects of alpha-chloralose. *Hum Toxicol* 1988; 7: 285–287.

Amitriptyline and related tricyclic antidepressants

Older tricyclics
Amitriptyline
Dothiepin
Doxepin
Imipramine
Nortriptyline
Protriptyline
Trimipramine

Newer tricyclics
Amoxapine
Lofepramine
Loxapine

Tetracyclic antidepressant
Maprotiline

General considerations

These drugs comprise one of the commonest groups of poisons encountered in clinical practice and are an important cause of poisoning deaths. They have marked anticholinergic actions, inhibit reuptake of catecholamines at peripheral nerve endings and have membrane-stabilizing effects. Tricyclic antidepressants are taken by about 12% of adults who poison themselves. Despite the advent of newer and possibly less toxic agents, amitriptyline and, to a lesser extent, doxepin and dothiepin predominate. Ingestion of 10 mg/kg body weight is likely to cause toxicity and 2.5 g or more is likely to be fatal, regardless of age. The toxicity of maprotiline, amoxapine and loxapine remains substantial but, in contrast, lofepramine seems considerably safer in overdosage.

Features

The major effects of tricyclic antidepressants are peripheral, on the CNS and cardiac.

Peripheral effects
These include warm, dry skin due to vasodilatation and inhibition of sweating, blurring of vision from paralysis of accommodation and pupillary dilatation and urinary retention.

CNS effects
Impairment of consciousness, respiratory depression and, less frequently, hypothermia are common. Coma is more commonly grade 2 or 3 than grade 4 and the lighter grades are associated with divergent strabismus, increased muscle tone, myoclonus, hyperreflexia, and extensor plantar responses. However, in very deep coma these features may be absent and it may be impossible to elicit plantar reflexes. Convulsions occur in a small proportion of cases during the early stages of intoxication but they are usually of short duration. Moving the patient or painful stimuli may provoke them and they, in turn, may precipitate cardiac arrest. Convulsions are more frequent after overdosage with maprotiline.

Cardiac effects
Tricyclic antidepressants have membrane-stabilizing actions. Hypotension is less frequent than with barbiturate poisoning causing comparable depression of consciousness and is due to a combination of dilatation of the venous capacitance bed, depression of myocardial contractility and occasionally, to extreme tachy- and bradydysrhythmias.

Conduction abnormalities are common in moderate to severe intoxication. The PR and QRS intervals are prolonged and the P wave may be lost in the preceding T wave. Second- and third-degree atrioventricular block are rare.

Sinus tachycardia due to vagal blockade occurs in over half the cases but important dysrhythmias occur in no more than 6% of cases.

Supraventricular and ventricular dysrhythmias (including torsade de pointes) occur in a small minority of patients and may be the cause of sudden deaths shortly after ingestion of the overdose. Paradoxically, bradycardia is present in some cases. The combination of sinus tachycardia with the conduction abnormalities indicated above often leads to a mistaken diagnosis of ventricular tachycardia.

Other features
Delirium and hallucinations may be present initially but consciousness is usually lost so rapidly as plasma concentrations of the drug increase that they are uncommon at this stage of intoxication. Urinary retention is common as are skin blisters. Rhabdomyolysis and subsequent renal failure may complicate overdosage with any tricyclic antidepressant but is a particular hazard with amoxapine and loxapine. Pneumonia and adult respiratory distress syndrome occur in a substantial proportion of patients.

Recovery-phase features

The recovery phase of tricyclic antidepressant poisoning is a twilight zone of impaired consciousness associated with restlessness and hallucinations. The patient continuously plucks at the bedclothes and commonly mutters to some relative who is not present. There is often considerable dysarthria, partly due to dryness of the mouth and tongue, and speech is extremely rapid, often of low volume and in-comprehensible. These features are normally accompanied by jerky, semipurposive movements of the eyes, head, limbs and trunk as if the patient is constantly being distracted by events in the environment, each competing for attention. The hallucinations are predominantly visual, taking the form of familiar people or objects, and are not usually as distressing as those of delirium tremens. The patient usually has complete amnesia for these events which may persist uninterrupted by sleep or sedation for 2–3 days. In some cases, however, the hallucinations are clearly frightening or there may be complete recall on recovery. During this phase the cardiac effects disappear in reverse order, usually within 12–24 hours.

Plasma concentrations of tricyclic antidepressants

Plasma concentrations of tricyclic antidepressants cannot be measured readily in hospital laboratories. Knowledge of them does not alter management and is unnecessary in the emergency situation. Limited studies in children show that concentrations below 500 µg/l are associated with anticholinergic features but not cardiac dysrhythmias or convulsions which tend to occur with concentrations above 1000 µg/l. Plasma concentrations do not correlate well with severity of toxicity in adults. They decline only slowly and this together with the fact that many of the major metabolites of tricyclic antidepressants are active may explain the late toxic effects.

Management

General measures
The stomach should be emptied if more than 4 mg/kg body weight has been taken within 4 hours of presentation or if the patient is unconscious. Coma should be managed in the conventional way, paying particular attention to the adequacy of ventilation.

Cardiac monitoring
Not every patient with tricyclic antidepressant poisoning requires cardiac monitoring or admission to an intensive care unit. Such resources are limited and should be reserved for patients who have evidence of cardiac toxicity and those who are unconscious or having convulsions since the latter commonly precede cardiac arrest. The duration of monitoring depends on clinical progress, bearing in mind that cardiotoxicity and seizures seldom present for the first time later than 24 hours after ingestion.

Convulsions
Avoidance of unnecessary stimulation of the patient may reduce the likelihood of convulsions occurring. If they do occur, however, they present a therapeutic dilemma. On the one hand they are usually short-lived, infrequent and resolve uneventfully. Suppressive treatment in these cases only further impairs consciousness and respiration. On the other hand, seizures are commonly the immediate precedent in the relatively small percentage of patients who have cardiac arrests. Despite this, it is doubtful if indiscriminate anticonvulsant therapy can be justified and they should be reserved for those in whom seizures are prolonged or recurring at short intervals. Intravenous diazepam is the drug of choice.

Cardiac dysrhythmias
The treatment of cardiac conduction abnormalities and dysrhythmias is controversial. Their aetiology is poorly understood and many doctors unrealistically expect them to respond to drugs used for similar problems complicating myocardial infarction. Antiarrhythmic drugs are themselves cardiac poisons and their indiscriminate use merely adds to the toxicological confusion. Conduction defects and dysrhythmias due

to anticholinergic compounds should not be 'treated' provided the patient is perfusing tissues adequately and is maintaining an acceptable blood pressure. Rapid intravenous infusion of sodium bicarbonate (1–3 mmol/kg body weight over 20 min) may be effective and should be tried before resorting to antiarrhythmic drugs. Occasionally, however, treatment for what appears to be ventricular tachycardia is necessary and lignocaine by cautious intravenous injection is the drug of choice. It has the merit of having a very short plasma half-life and will disappear rapidly from the circulation should it be ineffective.

Hypotension
Hypotension which cannot be attributed to extreme tachycardia or bradycardia should be managed in the conventional way.

Agitation, delirium and hallucinations
In some cases, agitation and restlessness are due to retention of urine and respond to appropriate corrective measures. Drug treatment of delirium and hallucinations may be necessary to alleviate distress and to reduce overactivity so that the patient does not injure him- or herself. Diazepam orally is adequate but large doses (up to 50 mg hourly) may be required initially to achieve the desired effect. Further doses are given according to the patient's condition.

Urinary retention
It is usually possible to empty a distended bladder by applying suprapubic pressure and catheterization should be avoided unless this is unsuccessful.

Measures to increase elimination
Tricyclic antidepressants have a very large volume of distribution and are eliminated by hepatic metabolism. As a consequence, forced diuresis, peritoneal dialysis, haemodialysis and charcoal haemoperfusion are ineffective. Repeated oral activated charcoal may be given but is of doubtful efficacy.

Physostigmine salicylate
The toxic effects of tricyclic antidepressants can be reversed by cholinesterase inhibitors such as physostigmine salicylate, a tertiary ammonium compound which is able to cross the blood–brain barrier. It is usually given in a dose of 2 mg intravenously over 2 minutes for an adult or 0.5 mg for a child. Within 5–10 minutes the heart rate slows and, depending on the initial depth of coma, consciousness may be regained or coma become less deep. Delirious, hallucinating patients given physostigmine rapidly become rational and lucid. Unfortunately

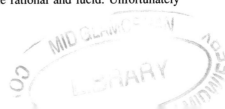

physostigmine is metabolized rapidly and its effects last no more than 30 minutes. This disadvantage could be overcome by giving repeated boluses or a constant infusion but there are other drawbacks to its use. It may precipitate convulsions, cause a troublesome increase in salivation and bronchial secretions and has been reported to cause ventricular tachycardia. Its role in the treatment of dysrhythmias is uncertain and, more importantly, there is no evidence that treatment with physostigmine is superior to supportive management. Its use has therefore largely been abandoned. Administration of physostigmine may be used as a diagnostic test for anticholinergic poisoning in cases where the cause of coma is in doubt. Its use is also justifiable in unconscious patients with serious respiratory complications in whom an early return of consciousness is desirable.

Prognosis

The outlook for patients who reach medical care is excellent but there is considerable dispute about what are the best early indicators of serious complications and outcome. For some years poisoning with a QRS interval of >100 ms was regarded as carrying an increased risk of convulsions and dysrhythmias but that view has recently been challenged. Statistical analysis suggests that the early features of poisoning, electrocardiographic changes and drug concentrations correlate poorly with the subsequent course of poisoning. Unconscious patients generally show significant improvement within 12 hours and regain consciousness within 36 hours. Cardiac conduction abnormalities and dysrhythmias usually resolve within 12 hours but delirium and hallucinations may persist for 2–3 days or even longer.

References

Dziukas LJ, Vohra J. Tricyclic antidepressant poisoning. *Med J Aust* 1991; **154**: 344–350.

Hulten B-A, Adams R, Askenasi R *et al*. Activated charcoal in tricyclic antidepressant poisoning. *Hum Toxicol* 1988; **7**: 307–310.

Lavoie FW, Gansert GG, Weiss RE. Value of initial ECG findings and plasma drug concentrations in cyclic antidepressant overdose. *Ann Emerg Med* 1990; **19**: 696–700.

Munger MA, Effron BA. Amoxapine cardiotoxicity. *Ann Emerg Med* 1988; **17**: 274–278.

Pellinen TJ, Farkkila M, Heikkila J *et al*. Electrocardiographic and clinical features of tricyclic antidepressant intoxication. *Ann Clin Res* 1987; **17**: 12–17.

Peverini R, Ashwal S, Petry E. Maprotiline overdose. *Am J Emerg Med* 1988; **6**: 247–249.

Reid F, Henry JA. Lofepramine overdosage. *Pharmacopsychiatry* 1990; **23**: 23–27.

Roy TM, Ossorio MA, Cipolla LM *et al.* Pulmonary complications after tricyclic antidepressant overdose. *Chest* 1989; **96**: 852–856.

Smilkstein MJ. As the pendulum swings: the saga of physostigmine. *J Emerg Med* 1991; **9**: 275–277.

Varnell RM, Godwin JD, Richardson ML *et al.* Adult respiratory distress syndrome from overdose of tricyclic antidepressants. *Radiology* 1989; **170**: 667–670.

Wolfe TR, Caravati EM, Rollins DE. Terminal 40-ms frontal plane QRS axis as a marker for tricyclic antidepressant overdose. *Ann Emerg Med* 1989; **18**: 348–341.

Angiotensin converting enzyme inhibitors

Captopril   Enalapril
                             Lisinopril

General considerations

Information on overdosage with angiotensin converting enzyme inhibitors is limited but indicates that it is an increasing problem. Fortunately, toxicity seems to be low. Healthy children also seem able to ingest up to 100 mg captopril or 30 mg enalapril without developing features. Similarly, single doses of up to 500 mg captopril, 300 mg enalapril and 400 mg lisinopril have been ingested by adults, resulting in plasma concentrations many times greater than those required to inhibit completely angiotensin converting enzyme, but did not cause serious problems. However, at least one death has been attributed to captopril.

Features

The only features of toxicity have been drowsiness (which may more probably have been due to other drugs ingested concomitantly), hypotension which was seldom severe and slight tachycardia. Although hyperkalaemia is a theoretical complication, it appears to be uncommon. No case of renal impairment has yet been reported.

Management

Until it is confirmed that the consequences of overdosage are minor and activated charcoal is effective, it is probably wise to empty the stomach if the overdose has been ingested within the preceding 4 hours. Hypotension is unlikely to require treatment but should it be necessary, intravenous saline is usually effective. Pressor agents should be necessary only rarely.

References

Dawson AH, Harvey D, Smith AJ *et al.* Lisinopril overdose. *Lancet* 1990; **335**: 487–488.

Park H, Purnell GV, Mirchandani HG. Suicide by captopril overdose. *Clin Chem* 1990; **28**: 379–382.

Spiller HA, Udicious TM, Muir S. Angiotensin converting enzyme inhibitor ingestion in children. *J Toxicol Clin Toxicol* 1989; **27**: 345–353.

Antibacterial agents

General considerations

Despite the wide availability of antibacterial agents in the community it is uncommon to encounter individuals who have poisoned themselves with these drugs. With the exception of antituberculosis drugs (considered separately), antibiotics are remarkably non-toxic in overdosage.

Features

The majority of patients will have no ill-effects. Occasionally transient nausea, vomiting and diarrhoea may occur. Single cases of renal failure after overdosage with co-trimoxazole, pancreatitis with erythromycin and haemorrhagic cystitis after amoxycillin have been reported.

Management

No specific treatment is required. Gastrointestinal upsets should be treated symptomatically if severe or prolonged. A good fluid intake should be encouraged.

References

Bright DA, Gaupp FB, Becker LJ *et al.* Amoxicillin overdose with gross hematuria. *West J Med* 1989; **150**: 698–699.

Goff D. Renal failure induced by co-trimoxazole. *Hosp Ther* 1989; **14**: 61–67.

Gumaste VV. Erythromycin-induced pancreatitis. *Am J Med* 1989; **86**: 725.

Anticholinergic drugs and plants

Anti-parkinsonian drugs
Amantidine
Benzhexol
Benztropine
Orphenadrine
Procyclidine

Mydriatic eye drops
Atropine
Cyclopentolate
Homatropine

Antispasmodic agents	*Plants*
Propantheline	*Atropa belladonna*
Mebeverine	*Datura* spp. (*arborea*
Oxybutynin	*candida, metel, rosei,*
Pipenzolate	*stramonium, suaveolens*)

General considerations

The drugs and plants listed above comprise only some of those with marked anticholinergic actions. Others include tricyclic antidepressants and the H_2-receptor antihistamines which are sufficiently important to be considered separately. Those discussed here may be accidentally ingested by young children who may also be attracted by the shiny black berries of *Atropa belladonna*, the deadly nightshade. Teenagers and young adults occasionally take anti-parkinsonian drugs or concoctions of parts of plants of the *Datura* species for 'kicks' (especially *Datura stramonium*, the Jimson weed, and *Datura suaveolens*, angel's trumpet). Of the drugs, orphenadrine is the most serious in overdosage and has caused deaths.

Features

The common features of anticholinergic poisoning have been summarized in one brief saying – 'red as a beet, hot as a hare, blind as a bat and mad as a wet hen' – which refers to peripheral vasodilatation, paralysis of ocular accommodation and the hallucinogenic effects on the brain. These are discussed in greater detail under amitriptyline. Coma, convulsions and cardiac dysrhythmias are rare.

Management

Management is as for amitriptyline (p. 68).

References

Danze LK, Langdorf MI. Reversal of orphenadrine-induced ventricular tachycardia with physostigmine. *J Emerg Med* 1991; **9**: 453–457.

Fahy A, Arnold P, Curry SC *et al*. Serial serum drug concentrations and prolonged anticholinergic toxicity after benztropine (Cogentin) overdose. *Am J Emerg Med* 1989; **7**: 199–202.

Furlanut M, Bettio D, Bertin I *et al*. Orphenadrine serum levels in a poisoned patient. *Hum Toxicol* 1985; **4**: 331–333.

Hildago HA, Mowers RM. Anticholinergic drug abuse. *DICP Ann Pharmacother* 1990; **24**: 40–41.

Snoey ER, Bessen HA. Acute psychosis after amantidine overdose. *Ann Emerg Med* 1990; **19**: 668–670.

Wells BG, Marken PA, Rickman LA *et al*. Characterizing anticholinergic abuse in community health. *J Clin Psychopharmacol* 1989; **9**: 431–435.

Baclofen

General considerations

Baclofen is used to reduce muscle tone in conditions associated with spasticity. Acute overdosage has usually been by ingestion and due to self-poisoning but the increasing use of continuous intrathecal infusion has led to intoxication from therapeutic misadventure. The consequences of poisoning are serious and deaths have been recorded. The plasma half-life of baclofen after massive overdosage has been reported to vary from 4.5 to 65.5 hours. The clinical course of poisoning is compatible with one of about 18–36 hours.

Features

The major effects are on the brain with impairment of consciousness leading to profound coma with hypotonia, hyporeflexia, hypothermia, hypotension and reduction of both the respiratory rate and tidal volume. Ventilatory failure and bradycardia are common features. First-degree atrioventricular block and QT prolongation were reported in one case.

The course of poisoning is measured over several days. Agitation, myoclonic jerks and convulsions have occurred during recovery from poisoning and occasional cases have been reported in whom the pulse rate and blood pressure suddenly increased for no apparent reason 48–72 hours after ingestion.

Management

There is no specific treatment for baclofen overdosage. The stomach should be emptied if the patient presents within 2 hours of ingestion or is unconscious. Management thereafter is supportive with particular attention to the airway, adequate ventilation and control of convulsions if appropriate. Atropine has been given for bradycardia and physostigmine for impaired consciousness following intrathecal overdosage; neither is a specific antidote. The effect of repeated oral activated charcoal has not been reported.

References

Lee T-H, Chen S-S, Su S-L et al. Baclofen intoxication: report of four cases and review of the literature. Clin Neuropharmacol 1992; **15**: 56–62.

Muller-Schwefe G, Penn RD. Physostigmine in the treatment of intrathecal baclofen overdose. J Neurosurg 1989; **71**: 273–275.

Barbiturates

Amylobarbitone	Pentobarbitone
Butobarbitone	Quinalbarbitone
Cyclobarbitone	Sodium amylobarbitone

General considerations

During the 1960s barbiturates were the most common drugs taken in overdosage and were responsible for a major proportion of poisoning deaths. Since then their role as hypnotics and sedatives has been largely supplanted by the benzodiazepines, and barbiturate overdosage is now relatively rare.

The former classification of barbiturates into short-, medium- and long-acting groups is inappropriate and misleading. The duration of coma after overdosage is comparable for all the barbiturates except phenobarbitone. The latter has a much longer duration of action which, together with other properties, is sufficiently important for it to be considered separately (see p. 195).

Features

The principal features of barbiturate poisoning result from generalized CNS depression. Drowsiness, ataxia and dysarthria are soon followed by coma, hypotension, respiratory depression and hypothermia. As coma deepens, the gag and cough reflexes disappear and breathing becomes shallow, though the respiratory rate remains normal or only slightly reduced. The pupils are neither constricted nor dilated but the limbs become hypotonic with loss of tendon reflexes. The plantar response, if present, is flexor but in deep coma may be absent. About 6% of patients develop skin blisters (p. 15).

Plasma barbiturate concentrations

Most clinical chemistry laboratories measure plasma barbiturate concentrations on an emergency basis but in general, they correlate poorly with the depth of coma, partly because of tolerance to the drugs and partly because of simultaneous ingestion of other CNS depressants, including ethanol. However, for any given grade of coma the plasma concentrations of cyclobarbitone and butobarbitone tend to be higher than those of amylobarbitone, pentobarbitone and quinalbarbitone. Concentrations after overdosage decline slowly initially, then more rapidly as enzyme induction develops acutely. Many texts refer to 'fatal' plasma barbiturate concentrations but it is not uncommon to encounter drug-tolerant patients who are awake and talking with plasma barbiturate concentrations well into the so-called lethal range.

Emergency measurement of plasma barbiturate concentrations is seldom justified since the result rarely alters management.

Management

Repeated doses of activated charcoal should be given. There is little merit in attempting to empty the stomach unless the procedure can be completed within 2 hours of ingestion or the patient is unconscious. Coma and skin bullae are managed conventionally.

The axiom that treatment should be determined by the patient's clinical state rather than the plasma drug concentration was never more true than in poisoning with barbiturate hypnotics. All but a small minority of those who reach hospital survive with careful, undramatic support of vital functions alone. Forced diuresis, peritoneal dialysis and haemodialysis intended to increase elimination of barbiturates from the body are potentially hazardous and largely inefficient. Those patients who are desperately ill, in deep coma with severe hypotension, respiratory complications, or who deteriorate or fail to improve despite intensive care should be treated by charcoal haemoperfusion. At present this is the method of choice for increasing elimination of barbiturates from the body but only patients satisfying the criteria on p. 51 should be treated in this way.

Prognosis

The great majority of deaths from barbiturate poisoning occur outside hospital and before medical care is possible. It is widely stated that the hospital mortality is less than 1% but most surveys claiming this degree of success include many patients with mild intoxication who were never at risk in the first place. The mortality increases with increasing depth of coma and is probably of the order of 5% in grade 4 coma despite high standards of supportive care. Death usually results from shock, cerebral oedema and respiratory infections.

References

Bismuth C, Conso F, Wattel F et al. Coated activated charcoal hemoperfusion. Vet Hum Toxicol 1979; 21: 81–83.

McCarron MM, Schulze BW, Walberg CB et al. Short-acting barbiturate overdosage. JAMA 1982; 248: 55–61.

Batteries (disc or button types)

General considerations

The widespread use of disc or button batteries in toys, electronic calculators, watches, hearing aids and a variety of other gadgets commonly found in homes has been accompanied by increasing numbers of children swallowing them. They cause damage in several ways:

1 The larger ones (diameters vary from 6 to 25 mm) may become stuck in narrow regions of the gut – the oesophagus at the level of the cricopharyngeus muscle and aortic arch are the usual sites.
2 They produce electrical burns of the gut mucosa if they were not fully discharged prior to being swallowed.
3 Leakage of their constituent chemicals may cause corrosive damage.
4 Systemic toxicity may develop if their constituent chemicals are absorbed.

The chemicals in disc batteries vary. Some contain mercuric oxide or silver oxide as their main constituent while others contain predominantly manganese dioxide. Varying amounts of concentrated potassium hydroxide are present in most types. Mercury cells seem to cause most problems, possibly because mercury oxide is itself corrosive, in addition to the concentrated alkali present and the mercury may be absorbed. Corrosive damage from leakage and electrical injury are considered to be closely related since although one may occur without the other, local electrical currents aid disruption of the seal between the two halves of the casing and therefore allow the contents to leak. The corollary of this theory is that intact discharged cells are unlikely to cause symptoms other than those attributable to impaction.

It is estimated that about 14% of batteries are themselves corroded as they pass through the gut. Mercury cells in gastric juice start to leak after about 24 hours.

Features

Only 10–20% of battery swallowers develop symptoms. Disc batteries which are greater than 15 mm in diameter are likely to stick in the oesophagus leading to retrosternal discomfort, difficulty in swallowing, cough, nausea and vomiting. Epigastric pain, haematemesis, diarrhoea and melaena may develop when the gut mucosa has been damaged, usually 24 hours or longer after ingestion.

Batteries lodged in the oesophagus may cause perforation leading to pneumothorax, mediastinitis, tracheo-oesophageal fistulae and, rarely, erode into the aorta causing catastrophic haemorrhage. Corrosive damage may also occur further down the gastrointestinal tract but rarely with the life-threatening consequences of impaction in the oesophagus.

Elevated serum mercury concentrations may be detected but, although the mercury content of a single cell comprises a potentially fatal amount for an adult, features of mercury toxicity do not occur.

It is estimated that corrosive features and/or increased mercury levels occur in about 10% of cases.

Management

General
It is helpful, but not essential, to try to identify the type of battery ingested by obtaining one similar to it and contacting the poisons information services who should be able to tell its chemical type from the code number engraved on it. Involvement of a mercury cell should increase awareness of the possibility of more serious effects. It is also useful to try to find out if the battery was new or spent since the latter are unlikely to cause problems.

X-ray the chest in every case to ensure that asymptomatic impaction of a battery in the oesophagus is not missed. A plain abdominal radiograph may make it possible to locate the position of the battery more precisely, indicate if it is leaking and aid further management.

Batteries stuck in the oesophagus
Batteries stuck in the oesophagus must be removed immediately. Open surgery should not be necessary; they can usually be removed by endoscopic techniques. Blind removal is not recommended. One of the most popular methods is to pass a Foley catheter beyond the battery, inflate the balloon and gently withdraw the catheter with the balloon still inflated, pushing the battery in front of it. A similar technique involves retrieving the battery by passing a cylindrical magnet down the oesophagus.

Batteries in the stomach
There is general agreement that leaking batteries in the stomach should be removed, as should those which are intact but have been retained for several days and are causing symptoms. Gastrostomy should be reserved for those patients in whom endoscopic attempts at removal have been unsuccessful.

There is doubt as to how aggressively intact batteries in the stomach should be tackled if they are not causing symptoms. For the following reasons a good case can be made for not intervening:

1 Most will pass through the pylorus without difficulty and only those retained in the stomach for 24 hours or more are likely to cause features.
2 Gastric lavage and induced emesis are ineffectual methods of trying to retrieve them.
3 Metoclopramide and laxatives have been used to shorten transit times through the gut but there is no evidence that they are effective and neither is without adverse effects.
4 Endoscopic techniques employing magnets offer the best chance of retrieval but the published success rate is no better than 50%.

Batteries in the small and large intestines
Batteries in these locations seldom cause serious symptoms and can generally be left to pass through the gut. About 90% will do so within 4–7 days although others take up to 4 weeks. Even when one seems stuck in one position for several days, removal is unnecessary provided the battery remains intact. As always, leaking batteries should be removed. Whole-bowel irrigation has been used successfully and should be attempted before resorting to open surgery.

Mercury toxicity
Elevated serum mercury concentrations are not uncommon after button battery ingestion and it is usually recommended that they should be measured if this type of cell has leaked in the gut. However, systemic poisoning is rare and older chelating agents have serious adverse effects which prohibit recommending their indiscriminate use. It is doubtful if they are indicated.

Reference

Thompson N, Lowe-Ponsford F, Mant TGK *et al.* Button battery ingestion: a review. *Adv Drug React Acute Pois Rev* 1990; **9**: 157–182.

Benzodiazepines

Alprazolam
Bromazepam
Chlorazepate
Chlordiazepoxide
Clobazam
Clonazepam
Diazepam
Flunitrazepam
Flurazepam
Ketazolam
Loprazolam
Lorazolam
Lormetazepam
Medazepam
Nitrazepam
Oxazepam
Temazepam
Triazolam

General considerations

The benzodiazepines were introduced in the early 1960s and have since been prescribed on a vast scale. They are now involved in about 20–40% of drug overdoses in developed countries. The use of benzodiazepines, and consequently benzodiazepine poisoning, is more common among women than men, probably because they are socially more acceptable than alcohol, which is the 'tranquillizer' preferred by men.

In general, benzodiazepines are remarkably safe in overdosage. Most young adults can ingest 30–40 or even more therapeutic doses without developing more than minor CNS depression. However, the elderly and those with chronic obstructive airways disease may be more seriously affected and there are now well-documented deaths from overdosage. Clinical impression suggests that flurazepam, flunitrazepam and triazolam are more dangerous. In addition, benzodiazepines are important because they potentiate the toxicity of other CNS depressants taken simultaneously and, when taken long-term, produce psychological and physical dependence. Most are metabolized to psychoactive derivatives.

Benzodiazepines taken alone
All benzodiazepines produce similar effects. When taken alone, they cause drowsiness, apathy, ataxia, dysarthria, partial ptosis and nystagmus. Coma, seldom deeper than grade 2 and lasting less than 24 hours, may follow. There may be mild hypotension and respiratory depression. Though they have been shown to exacerbate hypoxia and hypercapnia in patients with chronic obstructive airways disease, this rarely causes serious problems. Bullous skin lesions have been reported. The great majority of patients poisoned with benzodiazepines alone recover considerably within 24 hours. It must be remembered that many of these drugs have active metabolites with long plasma half-lives so that performance in skilled tasks (e.g. driving motor vehicles) may be impaired for several days or weeks after apparent recovery from the overdose and patients should be warned accordingly.

Benzodiazepines taken with other drugs
Benzodiazepines are commonly taken in overdosage with other psychotropic drugs and potentiate their CNS depressant effects. However, when taken with tricyclic antidepressants, there may be advantages in the combination since the anticonvulsant properties of benzodiazepines may prevent convulsions and help control delirium and hallucinations.

Management

General

Commonly, the toxic effects of benzodiazepines taken alone are so minimal that little treatment is required. Emptying the stomach is probably valueless. Repeated doses of oral activated charcoal have been recommended but seem superfluous in the context of generally low toxicity. Impairment of consciousness and hypotension should be treated conventionally. Rarely, endotracheal intubation and assisted ventilation may be required.

Flumazenil

Actions. Flumazenil is a specific benzodiazepine antagonist, capable of reversing serious toxicity due to these drugs within a minute. Its use is unnecessary in the great majority of cases and it should be reserved for patients who are seriously poisoned with deep coma and in need of endotracheal intubation or assisted ventilation, although it is not an alternative to supportive care. Some countries have not yet licensed flumazenil for use in benzodiazepine overdosage, although many reports testify to its value.

Dosage. Adults should be given 0.2 mg intravenously over 30 seconds. If consciousness is not regained within 30 seconds, 0.3 mg may then be given over the same period of time. Subsequent doses of 0.5 mg at one minute intervals are indicated if there is no response but it is doubtful if giving a total of more than 3 mg flumazenil has any merit; 1–3 mg is usually enough to reverse coma caused by benzodiazepines. If, and only if, 3 mg produces a definite but incomplete improvement, can further doses to a total of 5 mg be justified. Failure to respond to 5 mg flumazenil over 5 minutes virtually excludes benzodiazepines as a cause of CNS depression.

Duration of action. Like naloxone, the half-life of flumazenil is considerably shorter (about an hour) than that of the commonly encountered benzodiazepines and patients must be observed for relapse into CNS depression after initial reversal. In such cases, an intravenous infusion of 2 mg/hour may be given together with additional bolus doses as required.

Adverse effects. Complications of its use include convulsions, bradycardia, ventricular dysrhythmias and complete heart block. It has been suggested that the risk of these can be minimized by flumazenil only being given in titrated doses, by experienced persons and only after hypoxia, severe hypotension and dysrhythmias have been corrected. It should be used with caution, if at all, in patients with a history of convulsions, twitching, toxin-induced cardiotoxicity or who have ingested large doses of tricyclic antidepressants.

References

Geller E, Crome P, Schaller MD *et al*. Risks and benefits of therapy with flumazenil (Anexate) in mixed drug intoxications. *Eur Neurol* 1991; **31**: 241–250.

Herd B, Clarke F. Complete heart block after flumazenil. *Hum Exp Toxicol* 1991; **10**: 289.

Hojer J, Baehrendtz S, Gustafsson L. Benzodiazepine poisoning: experience of 702 admissions to an intensive care unit during a 14-year period. *J Intern Med* 1989; **226**: 117–122.

Leykin Y, Halpern P, Silbiger A *et al*. Acute poisoning treated in the intensive care unit: a case series. *Isr J Med Sci* 1989; **25**: 98–102.

Pulce C, Mollon P, Pham E *et al*. Acute poisonings with ethyle loflazepate, flunitrazepam, prazepam and triazolam in children. *Vet Hum Toxicol* 1992; **34**: 141–143.

Roald OK, Dahl V. Flunitrazepam intoxication in a child successfully treated with the benzodiazepine antagonist flumazenil. *Crit Care Med* 1989; **17**: 1355–1356.

Beta-adrenoceptor blocking drugs

Acebutalol

Atenolol

Labetalol

Metoprolol

Nadolol

Oxprenolol

Pindolol

Propranolol

Sotalol

General considerations

Acute overdosage with beta-adrenoceptor blocking drugs has been reported relatively infrequently considering their widespread use for treatment of hypertension, dysrhythmias and ischaemic heart disease. Presumably this is because they are prescribed for patients who are older than the average of those prone to take drug overdoses. The plasma half-lives of propranolol and atenolol after overdosage are about 6 and 8 hours respectively.

Features

There is controversy about the toxicity of large overdoses of beta-adrenoceptor blockers. While some patients have apparently ingested massive doses without ill effects, the majority of reports indicate life-threatening consequences even in those with normal cardiovascular systems.

The features of beta-adrenoceptor blocker overdosage vary somewhat from one member of the group to another. The onset of symptoms may be extremely rapid. Pallor and ataxia progress to coma with peripheral circulatory failure and cold, clammy, cyanosed extremities. Profound bradycardia is usually present, particularly when propranolol and oxprenolol are involved, with a reduced or unrecordable blood pressure. Electrocardiograms may show that the bradycardia is sinus or nodal in origin but it may be difficult to identify P waves with certainty. There may be marked QRS prolongation and ST and T wave changes. Convulsions (especially with propranolol), respiratory arrest or asystolic cardiac arrest may occur at any moment. The plasma potassium may be raised. Ventricular tachyarrhythmias have been reported, particularly in association with sotalol overdosage, and may be of the torsade de pointes type. Rarely, acute renal failure may ensue.

Management

General
Repeated doses of oral activated charcoal should be given. Convulsions should not be treated if they are short-lived and infrequent. Severe bradycardia and hypotension may respond to atropine 3 mg intravenously (or 0.04 mg/kg body weight) which may be repeated if necessary. The heart rate and rhythm should be monitored continuously.

Glucagon
Glucagon is the treatment of choice for serious cardiotoxicity. It is thought to work by activating adenylcyclase by a mechanism which is not blocked by beta-blockers. A single bolus of 5–10 mg has dramatic effects on the pulse and blood pressure and vomiting may be induced. In severe poisoning the response to glucagon may be transient and an infusion of 4 mg/hour should be given and reduced gradually as the patient improves. When large quantities have to be given it is preferable to use a preparation of glucagon which does not contain phenol as a preservative, or to use 5% dextrose instead of the diluent provided.

Beta-adrenoceptor agonists
While beta-adrenoceptor agonists are the logical antidotes to poisoning with beta-blockers, their value is diminished by the time it takes to reach an effective dose with a minimum of risk. The dose must be titrated against the clinical response. An isoprenaline infusion may be set up and the rate of administration increased until the desired increase in pulse rate and blood pressure is achieved. Since the isoprenaline is in competition with the beta-blocker at receptor sites, very large amounts may have to be given. Failure to appreciate this may account for the early reports of isoprenaline 'resistance' in beta-blocker poisoning. Prenalterol has a greater safety margin than isoprenaline; 5 mg is an appropriate initial dose for an adult but dosage has to be titrated against response. Dobutamine is a suitable alternative to prenalterol if the latter is not available.

Other methods of circulatory support
Rarely, intra-aortic balloon pumps and extracorporeal circuits have been used to sustain an adequate cardiac output while awaiting metabolism and elimination of beta-blockers.

References

Agura ED, Wexler LF, Witzburg RA. Massive propranolol overdose. *Am J Med* 1986; **80**: 755–757.

Critchley JAJH, Ungar A. The management of acute poisoning due to β-adrenoceptor antagonists. *Med Toxicol* 1989; **4**: 32–45.

Ehgartner GR, Zelinka MA. Hemodynamic instability following intentional nadolol overdose. *Arch Intern Med* 1988; **148**: 801–802.

Freestone S, Thomas HM, Bhamra RK *et al.* Severe atenolol poisoning: treatment with prenalterol. *Hum Toxicol* 1986; **5**: 343–345.

McVey FK, Corke CF. Extracorporeal circulation in the management of massive propranolol overdose. *Anaesthesia* 1991; **46**: 744–746.

O'Mahony D, O'Leary P, Molloy MG. Severe oxprenolol poisoning: the importance of glucagon infusion. *Hum Exp Toxicol* 1990; **9**: 101–103.

Perrot D, Bui-Xuan B, Lang J *et al.* A case of sotalol poisoning with fatal outcome. *Clin Toxicol* 1988; **80**: 389–396.

Smit AJ, Mulder POM, de Jong PE *et al.* Acute renal failure after overdose of labetalol. *Br Med J* 1986; **80**: 1142.

Bleaches

General considerations

The active constituent of most household bleaches is sodium hypochlorite in concentrations up to 10%. Bleaches have a corrosive action due partly to the alkalinity of the solution and partly to the formation of hypochlorous acid and liberation of free chlorine when hypochlorite reacts with gastric acid. The chlorine may, in turn, be inhaled and cause respiratory symptoms. Poisoning with household bleaches is largely confined to children below the age of 5 years.

Features

The majority of children who accidentally ingest bleach do not develop symptoms, presumably because they take only small quantities. About 35% have nausea and/or vomiting and 20% irritation of the buccal mucosa. Ulceration of mucous membranes and abdominal pain are uncommon. In contrast, the deliberate ingestion of large quantities can be fatal due to oesophageal ulceration, perforation, haemorrhage, metabolic acidosis and shock. Acute respiratory obstruction due to laryngeal oedema may develop if chlorine liberated in the stomach is inhaled. Hypernatraemia and hyperchloraemia have been reported in an adult after ingestion of a large amount of bleach.

Management

Most patients require very little treatment. If only small amounts have been ingested it will be sufficient to give milk or antacids. The stomach should be emptied if a large quantity has been taken provided there is no evidence of corrosive oesophagitis or gastritis. If readily available, sodium thiosulphate may be left in the stomach to reduce any remaining hypochlorite. Electrolyte and acid–base abnormalities should be sought and corrected.

Severe poisoning with burns should be treated as for strong acids and alkalis (p. 108).

Reference

Ward MJ, Routledge PA. Hypernatraemia and hyperchloraemic acidosis after bleach ingestion. *Hum Toxicol* 1988; 7: 37–38.

Calcium channel blocking drugs

Diltiazem   Verapamil
                             Nifedipine

General considerations

Calcium channel blocking drugs are widely used in the treatment of angina of effort and supraventricular dysrhythmias. They depress the sinoatrial and atrioventricular nodes and inhibit insulin release.

Acute overdosage with these drugs is uncommon but may be fatal. Most available information refers to diltiazem and verapamil which are rapidly absorbed from the gastrointestinal tract and extensively metabolized in the liver. The plasma half-life of diltiazem after overdosage is about 8 hours.

Features

The features of poisoning are normally apparent within 4 hours. The patient may be alert until a late stage. The predominant effects are on the heart with varying degrees of atrioventricular block leading to marked bradycardia with junctional escape rhythms and eventually asystole. As a consequence there is profound hypotension, peripheral circulatory failure and secondary metabolic acidosis. Hyperkalaemia and hypokalaemia have been reported, the former being commoner. Hyperglycaemia has been reported following overdosage with diltiazem and verapamil.

Management

The stomach should be emptied if the tablets have been ingested within 2 hours but the definitive treatment remains uncertain. Atropine may reverse the bradycardia and improve atrioventricular conduction. Calcium gluconate (adult dose 10–20 ml of a 10% solution given intravenously over 5–10 minutes under electrocardiogram control) has occasionally returned nodal rhythm to sinus rhythm but more usually it is ineffective. Cardiac pacing and inotropic support such as dopamine may be necessary. Plasma diltiazem concentrations of up to 4 mg/l have been reported after overdosage but the volume of distribution is large and techniques to enhance elimination are probably of little value. Hyperkalaemia (see p. 202) and hyperglycaemia may require appropriate treatment.

References

Erickson FC, Ling LJ, Grande GA *et al*. Diltiazem overdose: case report and review. *J Emerg Med* 1991; **9**: 357–366.

Ferner RE, Odemuyiwa O, Field AB *et al*. Pharmacokinetics and toxic effects of diltiazem in massive overdose. *Hum Toxicol* 1989; **8**: 497–499.

Ferner RE, Monkman S, Riley J *et al*. Pharmacokinetics and toxic effects of nifedipine in massive overdose. *Hum Exp Toxicol* 1990; **9**: 309–311.

Krick SE, Gums JG, Grauer K *et al*. Severe verapamil (sustained-release) overdose. *DICP Ann Pharmacother* 1990; **24**: 705–706.

Minella RA, Schulman DS. Fatal verapamil toxicity and hypokalemia. *Am Heart J* 1991; **121**: 1810–1812.

Ramoska EA, Spiller HA, Myers A. Calcium channel blocker toxicity. *Ann Emerg Med* 1990; **19**: 649–653.

Cannabis

General considerations

Cannabis, the Indian hemp plant (*Cannabis sativa*), contains several active constituents known as tetrahydrocannabinols. Cannabis resin (hashish) is obtained from the flowering top of the plant while the less potent leaves are termed marijuana, grass or pot. Cannabis is usually smoked or ingested but there have been occasional reports of intravenous injection of a 'tea' brewed from the plant. Very rarely intoxication may result from body packing.

Features

The effects of cannabis are more readily controlled if it is smoked rather than ingested. Using the former route symptoms start within 10–20 minutes and last about 3 hours while with the latter the onset may be delayed up to 2 hours and persist for up to 6 hours. The symptoms are very variable. Initially there may be mild anxiety and excitement followed by a feeling of calm, euphoria and uncontrollable laughter. Perception of colour and sound is often enhanced. Drowsiness and sleep follow. The only physical features may be an irritating, unproductive cough, dry mouth, tachycardia and conjunctival suffusion. On occasions, some individuals react with panic which may lead to hospital referral.

Intravenous injection of cannabis tea has much more serious consequences. Nausea, vomiting, abdominal pain and watery diarrhoea develop rapidly and are accompanied by rigors, fever, hypotension and shock. Renal impairment, cholestatic jaundice, muscle pain and weakness may become apparent over the next few days. The alterations in perception and cerebral function seen after cannabis has been smoked or ingested are strangely absent. A polymorph leucocytosis and thrombocytopenia may be found and hypoglycaemia has been reported. The electrocardiogram may show ischaemic changes.

Accidental ingestion of cannabis by children has caused coma with dilated pupils, hypotonia and hyporeflexia. Particles of cannabis may be found in the oropharynx.

Management

Treatment is usually unnecessary when cannabis has been inhaled or ingested but if consciousness is impaired, appropriate supportive measures should be used. Panic reactions usually respond to reassurance and sedation with diazepam. Intravenous fluids and symptomatic measures are all that can be offered to patients poisoned with· intravenous cannabis.

References

MacNab A, Anderson EA, Susak L. Ingestion of cannabis: a cause of coma in children. *Pediatr Emerg Care* 1989; **5**: 238–239.
Solomons K, Neppe VM. Cannabis – its clinical effects. *S Afr Med J* 1989; **76**: 102–104.

Carbamazepine

General considerations

Overdosage with carbamazepine appears to be increasing as its role as an anticonvulsant expands. Chemically and toxicologically, carbamazepine is similar to tricyclic antidepressants.

Features

Drowsiness, nystagmus, ataxia and incoordination are followed by loss of consciousness. The pupils are often dilated and divergent strabismus may be present during coma and disappear with recovery. Complete external ophthalmoplegia has been recorded. Muscle tone is often increased and opisthotonos and convulsions occur. When roused, patients tend to react violently and thrash around in bed. Choreiform movements and hallucinations may occur. Respiration is rarely depressed. Many of the adverse reactions to therapeutic doses of carbamazepine have not been reported after acute overdosage.

Management

Most patients should require nothing more than supportive measures. The plasma half-life of the drug after overdosage is considerably longer than with therapeutic doses and recovery is correspondingly slow. Repeated oral activated charcoal shortens the plasma half-life but there is doubt about whether patients recover more quickly as a result.

References

Durelli L, Massazza U, Cavallo R. Carbamazepine toxicity and poisoning. *Med Toxicol Adv Drug Exp* 1989; **4**: 95–107.
Wason S, Baker RC, Carolan P *et al*. Carbamazepine overdose – the effects of multiple dose activated charcoal. *Clin Toxicol* 1992; **30**: 39–48.

Carbon monoxide

General considerations

Carbon monoxide remains one of the most important causes of accidental and suicidal poisoning deaths. Smoke from fires is now probably the single most important source but car exhaust fumes and a variety of more subtle causes are also responsible. Many cases arise from the incomplete combustion of methane, butane and propane either because they have been used in a confined atmosphere (e.g. caravans) where ventilation may have been deliberately reduced to increase warmth or because the appliance is faulty or vents are blocked. The use of charcoal grills and paint removers containing methylene chloride in confined spaces has also caused carbon monoxide poisoning (see p. 152).

Carbon monoxide causes severe hypoxia by a number of means. It reduces the oxygen-carrying capacity of the blood by binding to haemoglobin to form carboxyhaemoglobin (the affinity of haemoglobin for carbon monoxide being 200–300 times greater than for oxygen), impairs oxygen delivery from the blood to tissues by shifting the oxyhaemoglobin dissociation curve to the left and prevents use of available oxygen by combining with cytochrome oxidases. These effects are compounded when other actions reduce cardiac output and tissue perfusion. It is therefore not surprising that morbidity and mortality should be high in elderly patients who have atherosclerosis.

In addition to acute poisoning, there is increasing concern over subacute and chronic intoxication.

Acute poisoning

Immediate features
The early features of carbon monoxide poisoning are headache, dizziness, nausea and vomiting. The vomitus may contain altered blood. Coma supervenes and is accompanied by hyperventilation, hypotension, increased muscle tone, hyperreflexia, clonus, extensor plantar responses, piloerection and shivering. Contrary to popular belief, the skin seldom shows the cherry-pink colour of carboxyhaemoglobin during life; a combination of central and peripheral cyanosis is much more likely. Skin blistering and rhabdomyolysis may occur if the patient has been lying for some time, but renal failure is very rare. Retinal haemorrhages and papilloedema secondary to hypoxic cerebral oedema may be present. Myocardial infarction, pulmonary oedema and a variety of neurological deficits such as mutism, parkinsonism, cortical blindness, hemiparesis and choreoathetosis have been reported. The latter correlate with lesions in the putamen and globus pallidus which can be demonstrated by computed tomography.

Arterial blood gas analysis usually shows a metabolic acidosis with a normal oxygen tension but reduced oxygen saturation and there may be electrocardiographic evidence of myocardial ischaemia.

Poisoning in pregnancy
Carbon monoxide intoxication during pregnancy is likely to cause miscarriage or premature labour. Fetal death is probably the result of severe hypoxia since the fetal oxyhaemoglobin dissociation curve, normally to the left of the maternal curve, will be further shifted to the left by the formation of fetal carboxyhaemoglobin.

Management

Supportive
The first steps are to remove the patient from the toxic atmosphere and ensure that the airway, ventilation and blood pressure are adequate. The oxygen concentration of the inspired air should be increased as far as possible. Any metabolic acidosis will usually respond to correction of hypoxia. Administration of alkali is best avoided since it will further

shift the oxyhaemoglobin dissociation curve to the left and impair oxygen release to tissues. Care should be taken not to give too much fluid intravenously, particularly in the elderly and in those whose electrocardiograms show ischaemic changes. Mannitol and dexamethasone should be given if cerebral oedema is present (p. 53). Assisted ventilation may occasionally be necessary in severe poisoning. The use of dantrolene should be considered if severe hypertonia is present.

Hyperbaric oxygen
Hyperbaric oxygen (HBO), first introduced for the treatment of carbon monoxide poisoning in the 1960s but discarded soon after, is again being used with enthusiasm. Protocols vary but often involve 2 hours or longer at a pressure of 2–3 atm. It has been advised for patients who have:

1 Been unconscious at any stage since exposure.
2 Carboxyhaemoglobin concentrations exceeding 40% at any time, regardless of the presence or absence of CNS features.
3 Neurological or psychiatric features.

The scientific rationale for this treatment is not in doubt since the half-life of carboxyhaemoglobin is of the order of 250 min breathing air, 50 min with 100% oxygen and 22 min with HBO at 2.4 atm. Despite this, there are uncertainties about its value in either reducing mortality or preventing long-term sequelae. The only controlled trial contained too few severely poisoned patients to reach a clear conclusion in respect of this critical group but showed that HBO was of no help to patients who did not lose consciousness (irrespective of their carboxyhaemoglobin concentrations - cf. point 2 above). These doubts, together with the relatively small number of hyperbaric chambers in some countries and the logistical difficulties of transporting sick patients to them, are considerable deterrents. Until the situation is clarified by further studies it seems reasonable not to refer patients for HBO unless they are unconscious or have very high carboxyhaemoglobin concentrations and the facility is readily available.

Prognosis
Most deaths occur in those who have sustained cardiorespiratory arrest at the scene or who are unconscious on arrival at hospital. Those who reach hospital alive are likely to survive.

Delayed features
More recently, there has been increasing awareness and concern over less well-defined neuropsychiatric sequelae of acute carbon monoxide

exposure. These develop in about 12% of victims, especially in those over the age of 40 years. About half the cases present 2–4 weeks after seemingly complete recovery and the remainder are equally divided between starting later and earlier. The features include lethargy, disorientation, inability to concentrate, recent memory impairment, hypokinesis, personality change as manifested by irritability, moodiness and a tendency to be aggressive and impulsive, and incontinence of urine and faeces. These abnormalities are considered to be due to lesions in the white matter of the brain.

About 80% of patients with delayed features will have returned to normal or be considerably improved within a year.

Subacute, chronic and occult poisoning

Subacute, chronic and occult carbon monoxide poisoning occurs in homes, commonly as a result of blocked flues and incomplete combustion of heating gases. The symptoms are vague and non-specific and a high index of suspicion is required if the correct diagnosis is to be made. Headache, dizziness, fatigue, general malaise and flu-like symptoms are the usual complaints and can clearly be due to many conditions other than carbon monoxide intoxication. The diagnosis often has legal implications and is best confirmed by demonstrating high carboxyhaemoglobin concentrations in the victims, bearing in mind that cigarette smokers may have levels of up to 8%. Room air should also be analysed to confirm leaks.

References

Crawford R, Campbell DGD, Ross J. Carbon monoxide poisoning in the home: recognition and treatment. *Br Med J* 1990; **301**: 977–979.

Peirce EC. Treating acidemia in carbon monoxide poisoning may be dangerous. *J Hyperbar Med* 1986; **1**: 87–97.

Proudfoot AT. Carbon monoxide poisoning – recent advances. *Acta Clin Belg* 1990; **45**: 61–69.

Raphael J-C, Elkharrat D, Jars-Guincestre M-C *et al.* Trial of normobaric and hyperbaric oxygen for acute carbon monoxide intoxication. *Lancet* 1989; **ii**: 414–419.

Shapiro AB, Maturen A, Herman G *et al.* Carbon monoxide and myonecrosis. *Vet Hum Toxicol* 1989; **31**: 136–137.

Ten Holter JBM, Schellens RLLAM. Dantrolene sodium for treatment of carbon monoxide poisoning. *Br Med J* 1988; **296**: 1172–1173.

Chloral hydrate and related hypnotics

Chloral hydrate   Triclofos
Chloral betaine

General considerations

Chloral hydrate is one of the oldest hypnotics. The other drugs listed above are rapidly broken down in the stomach to yield chloral hydrate and therefore have identical effects. Chloral hydrate is so rapidly metabolized by alcohol dehydrogenase to trichloroethanol that it is not present in significant quantities in plasma. Trichloroethanol is then oxidized to trichloroacetic acid. Poisoning with these compounds is uncommon. Chronic use may lead to physical and psychological dependence.

Features

Chloral hydrate irritates the oesophageal and gastric mucosae causing heartburn, nausea and vomiting. In other respects, however, most of the features of overdosage are similar to those of ethanol poisoning with coma, hypotension, vasodilatation and mild respiratory depression. The most serious complications are supraventricular and ventricular dysrhythmias leading to cardiac arrest. It has been estimated that ectopic beats should be expected in 25% of cases

Management

The great majority of cases will require no more than supportive care. Repeated doses of oral activated charcoal are indicated. Naloxone had no effect in one man who subsequently responded to flumazenil. The cardiac rhythm should be monitored but though dysrhythmias complicating chloral hydrate poisoning appear alarming, they often terminate spontaneously. If they cause haemodynamic problems, however, they respond dramatically to beta-blockade. Haemodialysis and haemoperfusion considerably shorten the plasma half-life of trichloroethanol, which is of the order of 13 hours after overdosage. However, they are only likely to be necessary in the rare patients who are very severely poisoned.

References

Buur T, Larsson R, Norlander B. Pharmacokinetics of chloral hydrate poisoning treated with hemodialysis and hemoperfusion. *Acta Med Scand* 1988; **223**: 268–274.

Graham SR, Day RO, Lee R *et al*. Overdose with chloral hydrate: a pharmacological and therapeutic review. *Med J Aust* 1988; **298**: 686–688.

Young JB, Vandermolen LA, Pratt CM. Torsade de pointes: an unusual manifestation of chloral hydrate poisoning. *Am Heart J* 1986; **112**: 181–184.

Chlorates

General considerations

Poisoning with chlorates is uncommon and is usually due to ingestion of sodium chlorate which is available as a weedkiller. Chlorates are powerful oxidizing agents.

Features

Chlorates irritate the gastrointestinal tract causing nausea, vomiting, diarrhoea and abdominal pain. Haematological effects, including intravascular haemolysis and methaemoglobinaemia, are common. As a result the blood may be chocolate-coloured and the plasma and urine dark. The patient will be cyanosed. Jaundice and oliguric renal failure may develop. A leucocytosis is common. Death may occur in the acute phase due to hypoxia secondary to severe methaemoglobinaemia or from hyperkalaemia.

Management

The stomach should be emptied if the patient presents within 4 hours of ingestion of the chlorate. Methaemoglobinaemia can be corrected by slow intravenous injection of methylene blue (0.1 ml of a 1% solution/ kg body weight), which may have to be repeated. Ascorbic acid is of no value. Blood transfusion may be necessary if there has been severe haemolysis but will be of limited value if chlorate is still present in the circulation.

The role of elimination procedures is uncertain. Haemodialysis will remove chlorate in severe poisoning and may be necessary for the management of renal failure. Plasmapheresis would be more logical in the early phase of poisoning since it can be used not only to remove chlorate, but also circulating free haemoglobin and red cell stroma which may predispose to the development of renal failure.

Chlorine

General considerations

Chlorine is widely used in industrial processes including water purification and the manufacture of hydrochloric acid, bleaches and plastics. Domestic exposure may occur if household bleaches are mixed with acidic lavatory cleaners or during school chemistry experiments. In addition to hydrochloric and hypochlorous acids, the reaction of chlorine with water produces several toxic unstable oxidizing agents. Inhalation of chlorine results in patchy necrosis of the respiratory mucosa at all levels and acute pulmonary oedema.

Features

Symptoms usually start within a few hours, the speed of onset being dependent on the magnitude of exposure. Lacrimation, conjunctivitis and cough are early symptoms and are followed by breathlessness, wheeze and expectoration of white frothy sputum which may become blood-stained. There may be hoarseness due to laryngeal oedema. Clinical examination usually reveals tachypnoea, and central cyanosis with crepitations and rhonchi throughout the lungs. Patchy and confluent areas of pulmonary oedema are present radiologically. Arterial blood gas analysis usually shows some degree of hypoxia and perhaps a metabolic acidosis but hypercapnia does not occur except at an advanced stage. A polymorph leucocytosis is common. Death is due to gross hypoxia and coma.

Management

The first step is to remove the patient from the toxic atmosphere. All but those who have been minimally exposed should be observed for 12 hours or advised to report immediately should they develop respiratory symptoms. The very young, elderly and those with preexisting respiratory disease are at special risk. Monitoring of the forced expiratory volume or peak flow rate will give early warning of deterioration. Oxygen therapy will be necessary if hypoxia is present. Bronchodilators may relieve bronchospasm but, since the pulmonary oedema is non-cardiac in aetiology, digoxin and diuretics are ineffective. Prednisolone 60 mg daily (or equivalent) should be given until symptoms have disappeared and there has been radiological clearing, then withdrawn over about 2 weeks. In severe cases, endotracheal intubation and assisted ventilation may be necessary if hypoxia cannot be adequately corrected by oxygen by face mask or if hypercapnia occurs.

References

Fleta J, Calvo C, Zuniga J et al. Intoxication of 76 children by chlorine gas. Hum Toxicol 1986; 5: 99–100.
Jones RN, Hughes JM, Glindmeyer H et al. Lung function after acute chlorine exposure. Am Rev Resp Dis 1986; 134: 1190–1195.

Chlormethiazole

General considerations

Chlormethiazole is a potent CNS depressant which is chemically related to vitamin B, and is used as a hypnotic and for the prevention of the alcohol withdrawal syndrome. Unfortunately it is frequently prescribed long-term to alcoholics who are continuing to drink. The practice is pointless and potentially dangerous since alcohol potentiates the CNS depressant effects of the drug and dependence on chlormethiazole commonly occurs. Chlormethiazole is extensively metabolized in the liver to inactive compounds, metabolism being impaired in the elderly and those with advanced cirrhosis.

Features

The features of chlormethiazole overdosage are similar to those of · barbiturate poisoning with impairment of consciousness leading to deep coma, hypotension, hypothermia and respiratory depression in severe cases. There is hypotonia, hyporeflexia and normal or absent plantar responses. The pupils do not show any specific changes. Increased salivation has been noted in a significant number of cases and may predispose to aspiration pneumonia. The smell of the drug may be apparent on the breath.

Management

Repeated doses of oral activated charcoal are indicated. Atropine may be given to counteract troublesome hypersalivation but is best avoided. Frequent pharyngeal suction and supportive care are all that is required for most cases. Forced diuresis would not be expected to be beneficial and haemoperfusion has been shown to be ineffective.

Plasma chlormethiazole concentrations

The limited data available suggest that plasma chlormethiazole concentrations correlate poorly with clinical assessment of the severity of poisoning and they are therefore of limited value in routine management. Patients with plasma concentrations up to 36 mg/l (about 20 times those after a single therapeutic dose) have recovered uneventfully. Coma is usual with concentrations above 7 mg/l. It should be noted that assays performed by ultraviolet spectrophotometry may be non-specific and give spuriously high plasma concentrations.

Reference

Ferner RE, Pottage A, Ryan DW *et al.* Charcoal-column haemoperfusion does not significantly enhance chlormethiazole removal. *Hum Toxicol* 1986; **5**: 367–368.

Chloroquine

General considerations

Chloroquine is a derivative of 4-aminoquinoline and is used for the prophylaxis and treatment of malaria and in connective tissue disorders such as rheumatoid arthritis and systemic lupus erythematosus. The considerable toxicity of this drug in overdosage is not widely appreciated; 300 mg proved fatal for a 12-month-old child and adults are unlikely to survive ingestion of more than 5 g.

Features

Chloroquine is rapidly and almost completely absorbed after ingestion and symptoms commonly start within an hour. Nausea, vomiting and drowsiness occur early and may be followed by slurring of speech, agitation, breathlessness due to pulmonary oedema, convulsions and coma. The most serious toxic effects are on the heart where the quinidine-like action causes hypotension, QRS widening, ventricular ectopic beats, ventricular tachycardia and fibrillation. The interval between ingestion and cardiac arrest may be as short as 3 hours or even considerably less. In one series 50% of patients who ingested 2.25 g or more of chloroquine base developed serious cardiac complications. Hypokalaemia is usual in severe poisoning.

Management

The stomach should be emptied if more than 250 mg has been ingested by a child or 1 g by an adult if they present within 2 hours. Give repeated oral activated charcoal. Hypoxia and acid–base disturbances should be sought and treated if necessary but hypokalaemia is best left uncorrected unless the patient is having multiple ventricular ectopic beats or torsade de pointes. Even in these cases, correction must be cautious because potentially lethal hyperkalaemia may develop as chloroquine is eliminated. Cardiac dysrhythmias should not be treated unless they are life-threatening since the administration of cardiac depressant anti-arrhythmic drugs to counteract the toxicity of another is illogical.

Diazepam reduces the morbidity and mortality from chloroquine intoxication but large doses have to be given (2 mg/kg body weight intravenously over 30 min) and endotracheal intubation and assisted ventilation are advisable before starting. The addition of adrenaline (0.25 µg/kg followed by increments of 0.25 µg/kg per min until a systolic pressure of 100 mmHg or greater is attained) further reduces mortality.

Tissue chloroquine concentrations are considerably higher than those in plasma and 70% of the drug is slowly excreted unchanged in the urine. It has been suggested, but not proved, that forced acid diuresis will increase elimination. Possible benefit from this treatment is extremely unlikely and must be weighed against the risk of pulmonary oedema in a patient with impaired myocardial contractility. There is no evidence that haemodialysis or haemoperfusion is useful.

Prognosis

Many patients severely poisoned with chloroquine are likely to have a cardiac arrest before reaching medical care. The absence of cardiac effects 4–6 hours after ingestion makes survival likely.

References

Jaeger A, Sauder P, Kopferschmitt J *et al*. Clinical features and management of poisoning due to antimalarial drugs. *Med Toxicol* 1987; **2**: 242–273.
Kelly JC, Wasserman GS, Bernard WD *et al*. Chloroquine poisoning in a child. *Ann Emerg Med* 1990; **19**: 47–50.
Riou B, Barriot P, Rimailho A *et al*. Treatment of severe chloroquine poisoning. *N Engl J Med* 1988; **318**: 1–6.

Chlorpropamide and related hypoglycaemic agents

Chlorpropamide   Gliquidone
Glibenclamide   Glyburide
Glicazide   Tolazamide
Glipizide   Tolbutamide

General considerations

Acute massive overdosage with oral hypoglycaemic agents appears to be rare. Most reported cases have involved chlorpropamide or glyburide (the latter being available in the USA but not in the UK) but the features of overdosage with other sulphonylureas is probably similar. These drugs stimulate insulin release from the pancreas and hyperinsulinaemia has been reported after overdosage. They also increase the pancreatic beta-cell response to glucose.

Chlorpropamide is particularly important within the group as a whole because of its very long plasma half-life (35–40 hours after therapeutic doses and probably much longer after overdosage). It is said to be rapidly absorbed but after overdosage peak plasma concentrations may not be attained for up to 39 hours. About 90% of chlorpropamide is protein-bound and approximately 80% is metabolized in the liver.

Features

The features of chlorpropamide overdosage are those of profound hypoglycaemia with impairment of consciousness, hypertonia, hyper-reflexia, clonus and extensor plantar responses. The pupils may or may not be dilated and convulsions may occur. Paradoxically the skin is usually dry. Because the plasma half-life of the drug is so long hypoglycaemia may be protracted or recur despite carbohydrate intake at any time up to 5 days after self-poisoning. Cerebral oedema, neurogenic diabetes insipidus, chronic vegetative states and death have resulted.

Management

Hypoglycaemia should be corrected urgently but even very large amounts of intravenous dextrose may not be sufficient to restore normal blood glucose concentrations or abolish the features of poisoning. Glucagon has been recommended if the patient presents within a few hours of ingestion but is unlikely to be effective after 24–36 hours because hepatic glycogen stores may have been depleted. Both glucose and glucagon will further stimulate insulin release and exacerbate the tendency to hypoglycaemia. Diazoxide is a more rational therapy as it blocks insulin release and raises plasma catecholamine concentrations. Intravenous therapy may be required initially (1.25 mg/kg body weight given over 1 hour) and repeated 6-hourly. Such doses do not cause hypotension. The plasma potassium will tend to fall and must be monitored carefully. Convulsions should respond to correction of the blood glucose but if this is not immediately possible, diazepam may be necessary. Cerebral oedema should be treated conventionally and repeated doses of oral activated charcoal given. Once the acute phase is over and provided repeated oral charcoal is not being used, diazoxide may be given orally (5 mg/kg body weight in two or three divided doses daily) until there is no risk of hypoglycaemia. Diazoxide causes sodium and water retention and care must be taken to avoid overload.

Elimination of chlorpropamide is enhanced by alkalinization of the urine but forced diuresis and haemodialysis are ineffective. Charcoal haemoperfusion removes significant quantities, shortens the half-life considerably and may therefore have a role in the management of very severe poisoning. Repeat-dose activated charcoal would be expected to be useful but has not been assessed.

There is no information on the use of elimination techniques in poisoning with other sulphonylureas but it is unlikely they would be required since these drugs have much shorter half-lives.

References

Erickson T, Arora A, Lebby TI *et al*. Acute oral hypoglycemic ingestions. *Vet Hum Toxicol* 1991; **33**: 256–258.

Ludwig SM, McKenzie J, Faiman C. Chlorpropamide overdose in renal failure: management with charcoal hemoperfusion. *Am J Kidney Dis* 1987; **10**: 457–460.

Mack RB. He is happy whom the muses love. Micronase (sulfonylurea) overdose. *NCMJ* 1989; **50**: 312–314.

Palatnick W, Meatherall RC, Tenenbein M. Clinical spectrum of sulfonylurea overdose and experience with diazoxide therapy. *Arch Intern Med* 1991; **151**: 1859–1862.

Cimetidine

General considerations

This drug is a histamine H_2-receptor antagonist which is used for the treatment of duodenal ulceration.

Features

Cimetidine is remarkably non-toxic in acute overdosage. Patients with plasma concentrations of cimetidine up to 57 mg/l (60 times the peak values obtained after one therapeutic dose) have been reported to have no symptoms other than drowsiness and dryness of the mouth.

Management

Treatment is unnecessary. A good urinary output should be ensured since cimetidine is excreted largely unchanged in the urine.

Reference

Krenzelok EP, Litovitz T, Lippold KP *et al*. Cimetidine toxicity: an assessment of 881 cases. *Ann Emerg Med* 1987; **16**: 1217–1221.

Clonidine

General considerations

Clonidine stimulates peripheral alpha-adrenergic receptors and also has CNS actions. Low-dose formulations are used for the treatment of migraine and menopausal flushing while higher-dose formulations are used in the management of hypertension. Poisoning is more common in children than adults and usually involves the low-dose preparation, probably because of its greater availability, attractive blue colour and sugar coating.

Features

Features usually develop within an hour of ingestion and seldom start or get worse after 4 hours. Drowsiness and impairment of consciousness are the commonest findings. The pupils may be constricted and unresponsive to light. Bradycardia is also common and hypotension is present in about 20% of cases. Much less frequently, severe hypertension occurs when peripheral effects predominate. Other features include pallor, apnoea, reduced respiratory rate, hypothermia, cardiac dysrhythmias and convulsions.

Management

There is no specific treatment for clonidine overdosage. Administration of emetics may be hazardous because consciousness may be lost rapidly and gastric lavage is the method of choice of emptying the stomach provided a clear airway can be maintained. Repeated oral activated charcoal is also indicated. Supportive measures, including assisted ventilation when necessary, are generally all that is required. The bradycardia usually responds to atropine. Naloxone has been used in attempts to reverse the CNS features but its value is uncertain and inconsistent. Alpha-adrenoceptor blocking drugs such as phentolamine and tolazoline have been shown experimentally to reverse the central and peripheral actions of clonidine but their value in human intoxication is unknown. They may, however, have a role in the management of severe poisoning, especially in the treatment of serious hypertension.

More than half the absorbed dose of clonidine is excreted unchanged in the urine in 24 hours but the value of forced diuresis and other measures intended to enhance elimination have not been critically assessed. They will seldom be indicated.

Prognosis

Considerable clinical improvement can be expected within 12 hours of ingestion and in most cases recovery will be complete within 48 hours.

Reference

Wiley JF, Wiley CC, Torrey SB *et al*. Clonidine poisoning in young children. *J Pediatr* 1990; **116**: 654–658.

Cocaine, amphetamines and related CNS stimulants

Cocaine
Cocaine hydrochloride
'Crack'
'Freebase' cocaine

Amphetamines
Amphetamine
Dexamphetamine
'Ecstasy'
Methylamphetamine

Related drugs
Caffeine
Diethylpropion
Fenfluramine

Pemoline
Phenylpropanolamine
Phentermine

General considerations

The occurrence of acute intoxication with cocaine, amphetamines and chemically related anorectic and stimulant drugs varies considerably from one part of the world to another, largely because it is most usually the result of their recreational use. It is therefore a problem of adults, although some cases of seizures in children have been caused by accidental ingestion of cocaine. In the last 10–15 years there has been a trend away from amphetamine abuse and towards cocaine as the latter has become much more widely available and cheaper. Poisoning is occasionally due to an acute overdose and is a hazard of body packing. More commonly, however, cocaine and amphetamine intoxication in particular are the result of the way in which the drugs are abused by addicts. The pleasurable effects of cocaine (and to a lesser extent amphetamines) decline rapidly despite its continuing presence in the blood so that 'binges' are necessary to maintain the effects. Repeated doses, occasionally as often as every 10 min or so for several hours, may be taken. Amphetamines are taken in a similar way but at less frequent intervals.

Cocaine is an alkaloid obtained from the leaves of the plant *Erythroxyum coca* and is usually available as the hydrochloride salt which is drawn up into the nostril for absorption or injected; it cannot be smoked. In contrast, 'free-base' cocaine and 'crack' (cocaine without the hydrochloride moiety) can be smoked, leading to rapid absorption through the lungs. Currently, the rapidly increasing use of 'ecstasy' is causing particular concern in the UK.

Features

The initial features of intoxication result from CNS stimulation. They include euphoria, talkativeness, restlessness, tachycardia, peripheral vasoconstriction, tachypnoea, tremor and dilated pupils. Nausea and vomiting may occur and facial flushing and sweating may also be present. As poisoning becomes worse, confusion, delirium, hallucinations, paranoia and violence towards oneself and others become prominent. The blood pressure may rise to extreme levels leading to a wide variety of serious CNS and cardiovascular complications, which are listed in Table 4.1. Hyperpyrexia, convulsions, metabolic acidosis, rhabdomyolysis and its complications may be fatal and, finally, consciousness and respiration may be impaired. Hepatic necrosis has also been described.

Table 4.1 Serious vascular, cardiac and neurologial complications of cocaine abuse

Dissection of the aorta	Subarachnoid haemorrhage
Myocarditis	Cerebral haemorrhage
Myocardial infarction	Cerebral infarction
Dilated cardiomyopathy	Cerebral vasculitis
Cerebrospinal fluid rhinorrhoea	Transient cerebral ischaemic attacks
Fungal infection of the brain	

Ecstasy is commonly taken by dancers in whom the high level of physical exertion predisposes to hyperpyrexia and rhabdomyolysis. Deaths have occurred and paranoid psychosis has been reported after 18 months of use.

Management

General
Repeated doses of oral activated charcoal should be given. Examination of the rectum or vagina is indicated if body packing is suspected and a plain X-ray of the abdomen may also be helpful in this context. Body packing should be managed as described on p. 43. Attention to the

airway and adequacy of ventilation are clearly imperative if consciousness is impaired. Arterial blood gas tensions should be measured and hypoxia and metabolic acidosis corrected as necessary.

Convulsions and agitation
Recurring convulsions should be managed in the usual way (p. 54). Patients who are agitated should be sedated with intravenous diazepam, particularly if motor activity is contributing to hyperpyrexia.

Haloperidol and similar drugs predispose to convulsions and are therefore best avoided. Dantrolene may be given if muscle tone remains greatly increased. Patients with these features, with or without hyperpyrexia, should be closely observed for the development of rhabdomyolysis and acute renal failure.

Hypertension
Hypertension should be reduced rapidly. Labetalol (intravenously at a rate of 2 mg/min according to response and to a total of no more than 200 mg) is preferred. Propranolol is best avoided as it has occasionally caused a paradoxical increase in blood pressure and the use of any beta-adrenoceptor blocker is contraindicated if the electrocardiogram shows evidence of ischaemia since they potentiate coronary vasoconstriction.

Dysrhythmias
Extreme tachycardia will respond to beta-adrenoceptor blockers. Other cardiac dysrhythmias should not be treated unless life-threatening, prolonged or recurring frequently.

Hyperpyrexia
Hyperpyrexia requires control of convulsions and reduction of muscle tone, as indicated above. Cold sponging may necessary but may be of limited effect due to toxin-induced vasoconstriction.

Elimination techniques
Forced acid diuresis was formerly advocated in poisoning with amphetamines and cocaine but is now generally held to be of little value and could be a serious risk in patients with hypertension and dysrhythmias.

References

Ernst AA, Sanders WM. Unexpected cocaine intoxication presenting as seizures in children. *Ann Emerg Med* 1989; **18**: 774–777.

Gawin FH, Ellinwood EH. Cocaine and other stimulants. *N Engl J Med* 1988; **318**: 1173–1182.

Hogya PT, Wolfson AB. Chronic cocaine abuse associated with dilated cardiomyopathy. *Am J Emerg Med* 1990; **8**: 203–204.

Hollander JE, Hoffman RS. Cocaine-induced myocardial infarction; an analysis and review of the literature. *J Emerg Med* 1992; **10**: 169–177.

Lange RA, Cigarroa RG, Flores ED *et al*. Potentiation of cocaine-induced vasoconstriction by beta-adrenergic blockade. *Ann Intern Med* 1990; **112**: 897–903.

Lessing MPA, Hyman NM. Intracranial haemorrhage caused by amphetamine abuse. *J R Soc Med* 1989; **82**: 766–767.

Loper KA. Clinical toxicology of cocaine. *Med Toxicol Adverse Drug Exp* 1989; **4**: 174–185.

McGuire P, Fahy T. Chronic paranoid psychosis after misuse of MDMA ('ecstasy'). *Br Med J* 1991; **302**: 697.

Nolte KB. Rhabdomyolysis associated with cocaine abuse. *Hum Pathol* 1991; **22**: 1141–1145.

Rubin RB, Neugarten J. Medical complications of cocaine: changes in pattern of use and spectrum of complications. *Clin Toxicol* 1992; **30**: 1–12.

Seaman ME. Acute cocaine abuse associated with cerebral infarction. *Ann Emerg Med* 1990; **19**: 34–37.

Shannon M. Clinical toxicity of cocaine adulterants. *Ann Emerg Med* 1988; **17**: 1243–1247.

Silva MO, Roth D, Reddy *et al*. Hepatic dysfunction accompanying acute cocaine intoxication. *J Hepatol* 1991; **12**: 312–315.

Sloan MA, Kittner SJ, Rigamonti D *et al*. Occurrence of stroke associated with use/abuse of drugs. *Neurology* 1991; **28**: 1358–1364.

Watson CJE, Thomson HJ, Johnston PS. Body-packing with amphetamines – an indication for surgery. *J R Soc Med* 1991; **84**: 311–312.

Colchicine

General considerations

Colchicine poisoning is uncommon and is usually the result of deliberate self-poisoning with colchicine tablets or ingestion of parts of the meadow saffron, *Colchicum autumnale*, though serious poisoning due to therapeutic misadventure has occurred. The mortality is high, particularly when the ingested dose exceeds 40 mg. Colchicine binds to tubulin, thereby preventing spindle formation and cell division.

Features

Symptoms usually start after 3–4 hours with vomiting, nausea, abdominal pain and diarrhoea, the latter being so profuse that the bowel motion resembles the rice-water stool of cholera. Bowel activity is reduced. Dehydration, oliguria, hypotension and shock follow rapidly. There may be burning in the throat with ulceration of the buccal mucosa. Muscle pain, tenderness and weakness, confusion, breathlessness (due to pulmonary oedema) and ventilatory failure often develop after 2–3 days.

Numerous laboratory abnormalities occur during severe colchicine poisoning. In some cases there is an initial polymorph leucocytosis but after as little as a few hours or as long as 4 days profound neutropenia and thrombocytopenia usually develop. As a result, severely poisoned patients usually die from infection and haemorrhagic complications. Mild hepatocellular damage and renal failure are common. The serum amylase may be elevated, though it is uncertain whether it is derived from pancreas or gut. Persistent hypokalaemia may be a problem and arterial blood gas analysis frequently shows a metabolic acidosis with hypoxia.

Paralytic ileus and convulsions have been described relatively late in the course of colchicine poisoning and alopecia does not usually become apparent till about 10 days after ingestion. By about the sixth day after poisoning the white cell and platelet counts begin to rise and may overshoot normal levels. Peripheral neuropathy is common in survivors.

Management

The uninformed physician may be lulled into an unjustified sense of security by the delay in onset of symptoms in colchicine poisoning. However, patients clearly require constant and prolonged supervision. The serious toxicity of colchicine justifies gastric lavage regardless of the number of tablets taken. Adequate intravenous fluids and electrolytes are essential at an early stage to replace gastrointestinal losses and maintain the blood pressure and urinary output. Unfortunately there is no method of enhancing the elimination of colchicine and reduction of mortality awaits the arrival of colchicine-specific antibodies which are currently being developed. Until then, complications must be sought and treated as they arise. Antibiotics and platelet transfusions may be necessary.

References

Davies HO, Hyland RH, Morgan CD et al. Massive overdose of colchicine. CMAJ 1988; **138**: 335–336.
Wells SR, Anderson DL, Thompson J. Colchicine toxicity: a case report. Vet Hum Toxicol 1989; **31**: 313–316.

Contraceptive preparations

General considerations

There are many different oral contraceptive preparations but most comprise a progestogen in combination with a synthetic oestrogen. They are virtually non-toxic.

Features

The majority of patients will have no symptoms. Nausea and vomiting may occur but settle rapidly. Vaginal withdrawal bleeding is a theoretical complication in prepubertal girls but seldom seems to occur.

Management

No treatment is required.

Corrosives

Strong acids
Hydrochloric acid
Nitric acid
Sulphuric acid

Strong alkalis
Ammonia
Lye
Potassium hydroxide
Sodium hydroxide

General considerations

Many poisons other than the strong acids and alkalis listed above have corrosive effects on the gastrointestinal tract but their other actions justify considering them separately. They include iron salts, paraquat, phenol, oxalic acid and mercuric chloride.

Poisoning with strong alkalis is uncommon in the UK but not infrequent in other parts of Europe and the USA where they are available for domestic use as drain, oven and pipe cleaners (particularly lye, a non-specific term for a mixture of sodium and potassium hydroxides). In consequence, accidental poisoning is most frequent in children, although accidental and deliberate self-poisoning in adults is not uncommon. Ingestion of strong acids is considerably less common and occasionally involves battery acid which contains dilute sulphuric acid.

It is thought that the titratable acidity or alkalinity of a product may be a better predictor of its corrosive potential than its pH. Strong alkalis are able to penetrate tissues deeply (including the eye) within less than a minute, producing liquefactive necrosis, whereas acids cause coagulative necrosis and penetrate tissues less well.

Features

Ingestion
The ingestion of strong acids and alkalis produces almost immediate burning pain in the lips, mouth, throat, substernal region and

epigastrium. Vomiting occurs very rapidly and may recur repeatedly with the vomitus becoming blood-stained. Hypersalivation is common. Shock and melaena may develop in severe poisoning. The patient may look pale and burns may be visible on the hands and face. A few patients escape buccal burns but most show red, oedematous areas with superficial desquamation. Only a small minority show deep destruction of buccal tissues but the larynx may be involved causing respiratory difficulties.

The development of oesophageal or gastric necrosis depends to some extent on whether an acid or alkali has been ingested. Alkalis commonly produce oesophageal burns but only about 20% of patients have gastric lesions. In contrast, the oesophageal mucosa is relatively resistant to acids whereas the gastric mucosa, particularly in the region of the antrum, is especially vulnerable.

Following alkali ingestion about a third of patients with mouth burns have similar lesions in the oesophagus. Oesophageal necrosis may be present in about 15% of those without buccal abnormalities. In severe cases the oesophagus may perforate leading to mediastinitis but this is more likely to be a complication of oesophagoscopy. The major long-term complication is oesophageal stricture formation and oesophageal carcinoma may develop at such sites after 20–30 years.

Gastric damage due to acids can be equally severe with haemorrhage, gangrene (which may involve the whole stomach) and peritonitis. Antral strictures usually become apparent 3 weeks to 3 months after ingestion or even much later.

Skin contact
Skin contact with strong corrosives may lead to burns of varying thickness with pain, blistering and ulceration.

Inhalation
Rarely, fumes from strongly corrosive agents are inhaled causing laryngeal and pulmonary oedema with corresponding respiratory symptoms. A pneumothorax occurred in one case.

Eye contamination
The severity of features following eye contamination by corrosives depends very much on the agent involved. They may vary from watering and irritation to redness and corneal oedema and ulceration. As with other tissues, strong alkalis (particularly those listed above) are able to penetrate the eye deeply and rapidly, raising the intraocular pressure and leading, in time, to cataract formation, uveitis and, rarely, retinal damage.

Management of ingestion of corrosives

General

Every case should be referred to hospital for assessment. Milk should he given as a first-aid measure to help neutralize the corrosive but in severe cases the patient is unlikely to be able to retain it. There is no merit in wasting time searching for citric acid, vinegar or sodium bicarbonate. Gastric emptying by any means is contraindicated. Analgesics and intravenous fluids or blood are often required and metabolic acidosis should be sought and treated appropriately. Oxygen and endotracheal intubation may be required if the larynx is involved. Management thereafter is controversial.

Corticosteroids

There is no convincing evidence in humans that administration of corticosteroids limits damage or prevents long-term sequelae.

Endoscopy

Upper alimentary endoscopy in the acute phase is hazardous but is necessary to exclude the presence of oesophageal burns so that hospitalization is no longer than necessary or to identify patients at risk of serious injury to the stomach or long-term sequelae. Those with deep circumferential oesophageal burns have about a 50% likelihood of having serious gastric damage and developing strictures.

Endoscopy should only be performed by an experienced endoscopist using a smaller instrument than usual. There is dispute as to how far the instrument should be passed. Some recommend that it should not be passed beyond the first burn since attempts to progress further are associated with a greatly increased incidence of perforation, while others maintain that minor burns are of little import but that the presence or absence of circumferential burns must be established. In some centres the stomach and duodenum are also inspected when possible.

Laparotomy

One study reported about a 50% incidence of gastric necrosis in patients with circumferential oesophageal burns and recommended laparotomy if the latter were found, damage being repaired as best it can. Since many of these patients also went on to develop oesophageal strictures, a string was placed so that guided dilatation of the oesophagus from below could be carried out if necessary.

Other measures

Patients with mediastinitis should, if possible, be managed conservatively. However, surgery, including resection, may be necessary if there is perforation or serious haemorrhage from the stomach.

Management of skin contamination by corrosives

Prolonged irrigation with water is indicated and other measures are indicated if the chemical involved is hydrofluoric acid (see p. 123). The cleaned lesions are then treated as burns.

Management of inhalation of corrosives

Maintenance of a clear airway is of prime importance and assessment of the extent of damage by fibreoptic endoscopy may be required. Observation is all that is required in asymptomatic patients and regular measurement of forced expiratory volume or peak respiratory flow rate may give warning of deterioration in function.

Management of eye contamination by corrosives

It is vital to start decontamination of the eye at the scene of the incident. The face should be submerged under water and the eye repeatedly opened and closed. Alternatively, tap water should be run into the eye. These measures should continue for at least 10–15 min.

On arrival at the emergency department, the conjunctival recesses should be carefully examined for the presence of particles which should be removed. Irrigation should continue using a 0.9% saline infusion directed to the eye through drip tubing. Repeated instillation of local anaesthetics such as amethocaine reduces patient distress and enables more thorough decontamination.

Corneal damage may be detected by instillation of fluorescein. Patients with such damage and those whose eyes have been exposed to any strong corrosive should be referred for expert ophthalmological assessment.

References

Anderson KD, Rouse TM, Randolph JG. A controlled trial of corticosteroids in children with corrosive injury of the esophagus. *N Engl J Med* 1990; **323**: 637–640.

Beare J. Management of chemical burns of the eye. In *Major Chemical Disasters – Medical Aspects of Management*, (Murray V, ed). London: Royal Society of Medicine Services, 1990, pp 157–167.

Herr RD, White GL, Bernhisel K *et al*. Clinical comparison of ocular irrigation fluids following chemical injury. *Am J Emerg Med* 1991; **9**: 228–231.

Isolauri J, Markkula H. Lye ingestion and carcinoma of the esophagus. *Acta Chir Scand* 1989; **155**: 269–271.

Knapp MJ, Bunn WB, Stave GM. Adult respiratory distress syndrome from sulfuric acid fume inhalation. *South Med J* 1991; **84**: 1031–1033.

Lorrette JJ, Wilkinson JA. Alkaline chemical burn to the face requiring full-thickness skin grafting. *Ann Emerg Med* 1988; **17**: 739–741.

Meredith JW, Kon ND, Thompson JN. Management of injuries from liquid lye ingestion. *J Trauma* 1988; **28**: 1173–1180.

Nash PE, Tacgakra SS, Baird H. Pneumothorax following inhalation of caustic soda fumes. *Arch Emerg Med* 1988; **5**: 45–47.

Sugawa C, Lucas CE. Caustic injury of the upper gastrointestinal tract in adults: a clinical and endoscopic study. *Surgery* 1989; **106**: 802–807.

Vergauwen P, Moulin D, Buts JP *et al*. Caustic burns of the upper digestive and respiratory tracts. *Eur J Pediatr* 1991; **150**: 700–703.

Cotoneaster

General considerations

Several varieties of this garden shrub and the related species, pyracantha, are cultivated in Europe and North America. During the autumn the plants carry numerous attractive scarlet berries which have a fleshy exterior and a central stone which contains the seeds. The seeds contain cyanogenic glycosides but it is highly improbable that a sufficient number would be eaten to cause serious symptoms.

Features

Most children will have no symptoms. Others may vomit or develop abdominal pain or diarrhoea.

Management

Treatment is usually superfluous. If a large number of berries has been ingested activated charcoal should be given. Symptomatic measures may rarely be required.

Cyanide

General considerations

Hydrocyanic acid is widely used in industry but with such stringent precautions that poisoning is extremely uncommon. Poisoning in industry is usually by skin contamination and/or inhalation. Sodium cyanide is used in less well-controlled circumstances for the elimination of colonies of rabbits and illegally to poison game fish in rivers. Hydrogen cyanide is produced in fires involving the decomposition of polyurethane foams and from the hydrolysis of laetrile (amygdalin), a cyanogenic glycoside contained in the kernels of apricots, cherries and other plants of the Rosacea family. Cyanide is readily absorbed by inhalation, through the skin and by ingestion. Cyanide poisoning may also result from ingestion of acetonitrile (methyl cyanide) used in beauty products (see p. 220).

The cyanide ion binds strongly to the ferric component of cytochrome oxidase, effectively preventing utilization of oxygen by cells and causing hypoxia. Anaerobic glycolysis and severe metabolic acidosis result.

Features

Most of the clinical features of cyanide poisoning are due to severe hypoxia although cyanosis is not present. The odour of bitter almonds on the breath is said to be characteristic but it is not always present and even if it were, it is questionable how many doctors would recognize it. Early symptoms of poisoning include feelings of anxiety, headache, dizziness, palpitations, weakness and drowsiness. Consciousness will be lost in severe cases and convulsions and cerebral oedema may be problems. Cardiorespiratory abnormalities may become prominent with breathlessness, tachypnoea, hypotension, pulmonary oedema, brady-cardia, conduction defects and dysrhythmias. Arterial blood gas analysis shows a metabolic acidosis.

Management

Preventing absorption
When hydrogen cyanide has been inhaled the patient must be removed from the toxic atmosphere, contaminated clothing removed and exposed skin thoroughly washed. When cyanide has been ingested, gastric aspiration and lavage should be carried out. The use of a 5% solution of sodium thiosulphate for lavage has been recommended but the procedure should not be delayed if this is not immediately available. Likewise 200 ml of 25% sodium thiosulphate may be left in the stomach at the end of lavage.

Supportive measures
The importance of supportive measures to establish and maintain a clear airway and ventilation cannot be emphasized too strongly. Oxygen in high concentrations must be given and metabolic acidosis should be sought and corrected. These measures may be sufficient to improve the blood pressure but the use of vasopressor agents is contraindicated because of their ability to cause dysrhythmias in the presence of hypoxia.

Antidotes
Contrary to popular belief, most patients do not die within minutes of cyanide poisoning. Indeed many survive severe poisoning for hours

before being given antidotes and others have recovered uneventfully with no more than the supportive therapy described above. These facts in no way belittle the importance of antidotes but merely emphasize that their role is complementary. Because the antidotes are potentially dangerous in the absence of cyanide ions the diagnosis must be beyond doubt before they are given and clinically the poisoning should be moderate or severe (i.e. with impairment of consciousness). The antidote of choice is dicobalt edetate (Kelocyanor) 600 mg intravenously. A further 300 mg may be given a few minutes later if the first dose does not produce a satisfactory response. The recommendation that it should be followed by 25 g of glucose intravenously is harmless but valueless.

If dicobalt edetate is not available the older intravenous regime of sodium nitrite (10 ml of a 3% solution given over 3 min) followed by sodium thiosulphate (50 ml of a 25% solution given over 10 min) should be used. For children the dose of nitrite should be 10 mg/kg immediately and 5 mg/kg after 30 min if necessary. Methaemoglobin produced by sodium nitrite binds cyanide ions avidly to form cyanmethaemoglobin and facilitates the transfer of cyanide bound to tissue cytochrome oxidases to haemoglobin where it is less harmful. Thiosulphate provides the sulphur to combine with cyanide via rhodanese to form non-toxic thiocyanate which is then excreted in the urine. The rationale of the first-aid measure involving the inhalation of amyl nitrite is similar but it is doubtful if sufficient methaemoglobin could be produced in this way without causing serious hypotension and it is not recommended.

References

Gonzales J, Sabatini S. Cyanide poisoning: pathophysiology and current approaches to therapy. *Int J Artific Organs* 1989; **12**: 347–355.

Johnson RP, Mellors JW. Arteriolization of venous blood gases: a clue to the diagnosis of cyanide poisoning. *J Emerg Med* 1988; **6**: 401–404.

Michaelis HC, Clemens C, Kijewski H *et al.* Acetonitrile serum concentrations and cyanide blood levels in a case of suicidal oral acetonitrile ingestion. *Clin Toxicol* 1991; **29**: 447–458.

Singh BM, Coles N, Lewis P *et al.* The metabolic effects of fatal cyanide poisoning. *Postgrad Med J* 1989; **65**: 923–925.

Dieffenbachia, Monstera and *Philodendron*

General considerations

Dieffenbachia, Monstera and *Philodendron* are members of the Araceae family of plants (frequently referred to as aroids) and are commonly grown throughout Europe and North America as ornamental house plants. They share a common mode of toxicity, though only the genus *Dieffenbachia* has been studied extensively. All parts of the plant contain specialized cells in which there are bundles (raphides) of needle-like crystals of calcium oxalate. When the plant is chewed the sharp crystals injure the mucous membrane allowing a proteolytic enzyme to penetrate. The latter is thought to be responsible for most of the ensuing inflammation.

Poisoning with these plants is most common in children.

Features

In practice, chewing the leaves or stems of these plants seldom seems to cause serious problems although it is commonly held to induce almost immediate, intense, burning pain in the lips and mouth and hyper-salivation. The buccal mucosa, lips, tongue and palate are said to become inflamed and swollen due to oedema making speech difficult or impossible. The latter has earned *Dieffenbachia* the popular name 'dumb cane'. In severe cases acute laryngeal oedema may develop and cause serious respiratory obstruction, especially in small children. Retrosternal pain and oesophageal necrosis have been reported in an adult.

The oedema usually subsides within 3 or 4 days but pain may persist longer.

Management

If required, treatment is symptomatic. Some relief may be obtained from sucking ice and milk or antacids have been recommended. Serious respiratory obstruction due to laryngeal oedema may require endotracheal intubation (if possible) or tracheostomy. Corticosteroids may be given but their value in settling the oedema has not been assessed.

Reference

Mrvos R, Dean BS, Krenzelok EP. *Philodendron/Dieffenbachia* ingestions: are they a problem? *Clin Toxicol* 1991; **29**: 485–491.

Digoxin and digitoxin

General considerations

While therapeutic intoxication with cardiac glycosides is common, acute massive overdosage is relatively rare, presumably reflecting the very small number of people needing these drugs in the age groups in which self-poisoning is most common. However acute digoxin and digitoxin poisoning occasionally occurs in children and adults whose hearts are normal. Overdosage is usually the result of ingestion but self-poisoning by the intravenous route has been described.

Rarely, poisoning with cardiac glycosides is due to ingestion of plants such as yew, Mediterranean oleander (*Nerium oleander*) and yellow oleander (*Thevetia peruviana*).

Digoxin poisoning has been reported from the UK, Scandinavia and North America while most accounts of digitoxin poisoning have come from the European continent.

Features

Nausea, vomiting, diarrhoea and extreme wretchedness are early features and drowsiness, confusion and delirium are not uncommon. Pale, cold extremities and hypotension indicate reduced cardiac output.

The most important toxic effects are on the heart. It is generally accepted that membrane adenosine triphosphatase is inhibited with resultant increase in intracellular sodium concentrations and leakage of potassium from the cells. Hyperkalaemia is common in severe cases. In the early stages of poisoning the loss of intracellular potassium reduces the resting membrane potential and increases the excitability of the myocardium. However, if the membrane potential is further reduced by continuing potassium leakage, excitability is impaired since the rapid inflow phase of the action potential is diminished in proportion to the resting membrane potential.

Sinus arrest and sinoatrial block are occasionally encountered but the commonest problem is sinus bradycardia with PR prolongation progressing to varying degrees of atrioventricular block and atrioventricular dissociation. As a consequence junctional escape rhythms may develop. His bundle electrography has shown that the block occurs in the atrioventricular node but there is dispute about slowing of conduction in the bundle of His and the Purkinje system. Though ventricular ectopics, bigeminy, ventricular tachycardia and paroxysmal atrial tachycardia may occur, the evidence suggests that they are more frequent with therapeutic intoxication than in acute overdosage in patients with normal hearts.

In addition to hyperkalaemia there may be hypoxia and a metabolic acidosis due to impaired tissue perfusion.

Management

Supportive
Oral activated charcoal should be given to interrupt enterohepatic circulation of the drug and given repeatedly until signs of serious

toxicity have passed. The latter is more important with digitoxin than digoxin. Cholestyramine (4 g orally four times daily for an adult) or colestipol, a steroid-binding resin (5 g orally four times daily for an adult) may be used as alternatives to charcoal.

The plasma potassium and urea should be measured urgently and hyperkalaemia (>6.0 mmol/l) treated as described on p. 202. Arterial blood gas analysis is advised if there is any suspicion of impaired tissue perfusion and hypoxia and metabolic acidosis corrected appropriately.

The cardiac rhythm must be monitored continuously. Sinus brady-cardia, ventricular ectopics, atrioventricular block and sinoatrial stand-still or block are often reduced or abolished by atropine (1.2 mg intravenously as required). Ventricular ectopics alone should not be treated unless cardiac output is impaired. Cardiac dysrhythmias should be managed conventionally, at least initially, though treatment with digoxin-specific antibodies may be indicated (see below). Direct current countershock should be avoided if at all possible.

Failure to achieve a satisfactory cardiac output by drug therapy in patients with bradycardia, atrioventricular block or sinus arrest is an indication for insertion of a right ventricular pacing catheter. It has also been suggested that this should be done prophylactically if severe hyperkalaemia is present since this may presage the onset of serious bradydysrhythmias. The pacing threshold tends to rise with increasing severity of poisoning and in the worst cases pacing may fail to initiate contraction.

Digoxin-specific antibodies
Severe intoxication with cardiac glycosides (as evidenced by ventricular tachydysrhythmias and peripheral circulatory failure) is an indication for treatment with Fab fragments of digoxin antibodies. They also cross-react with digitoxin and lanatoside C. Their use rapidly produces return of sinus rhythm, correction of hyperkalaemia and decline in plasma concentrations of free digoxin over about 4 hours. The dose required depends on the total body load of glycoside.

To estimate the total body load of a cardiac glycoside (for a patient not previously on treatment with the drug), either:

1   multiply the amount ingested (in mg) by 0.8 to allow for the bioavailability of the drug; or
2 (a) multiply the plasma digoxin concentration (in ng/ml) by 5.6 (the volume of distribution of the drug in an average adult), then
  (b) multiply the figure obtained by the weight of the patient, then
  (c) finally divide the figure obtained in 2(b) by 1000 to obtain the body load (in mg).

When acute overdosage is superimposed on therapeutic doses of the glycoside, the total body load is the sum of the figures obtained by both of these.

The dose of Fab fragments (in mg) is found by multiplying the body load of digoxin by 64.

Elimination techniques

Elimination techniques have no role in the management of poisoning with cardiac glycosides. Most of the drug is tissue-bound, the volume of distribution is large, plasma concentrations are low and toxicologically significant amounts of the drug cannot be removed. Digoxin is excreted through the kidneys but forced diuresis does not increase its clearance except in the first 4–6 hours after a large overdose before distribution of the drug has been completed. Even in these optimal circumstances, however, only very small quantities of drug can be recovered. Exchange transfusion, peritoneal dialysis and haemodialysis are of no value and, though claims have been made for the usefulness of charcoal and resin haemoperfusion, adequate confirmatory data are lacking.

Prognosis

Acute digoxin overdosage formerly carried a mortality of 10–20% but this should be greatly reduced by the use of digoxin antibodies. However, success depends on administration before patients become moribund and on the severity of underlying heart disease, if present.

References

Antman EM, Wenger TL, Butler VP *et al.* Treatment of 150 cases of life-threatening digitalis intoxication with digoxin-specific Fab antibody fragments. *Circulation* 1990; **81**: 1744–1752.

Banner W, Bayer MJ, Smith TW (eds). Digitalis intoxication. Update on clinical recognition and management. *Ann Emerg Med* 1991; **9**: supplement 1.

Cheung K, Hinds JA, Duffy P. Detection of poisoning by plant-origin glycoside with the Abbott TDx analyser. *Clin Chem* 1989; **35**: 295–297.

Disinfectants

General considerations

Serious poisoning with household disinfectants is now uncommon compared with some decades ago when Lysol (50% cresol) was frequently used in suicide attempts. The active constituent of most present-day liquid disinfectants is dichlorometaxylenol (DCMX). Others contain pine oil and chlorhexidine and there are still some which have phenol (carbolic acid) or cresol (methylphenol) as the active ingredient. In addition they contain miscellaneous other ingredients including soaps, castor oil and isopropanol which vary from one brand to another and add significantly to the toxicity when large volumes are ingested. There is considerable knowledge about the toxic effects of phenol and cresol (which for practical purposes are identical). Information about DCMX is very limited but it probably causes similar harm.

Features

Ingestion of large quantities of any of the active ingredients causes burns of the lips, mouth and upper alimentary tract but, with the exception of phenolic substances, the lesions are usually mild. However, laryngeal involvement is a potential cause of hoarseness, stridor and acute respiratory obstruction.

Pine oil-based products may also cause ataxia and CNS depression varying from drowsiness to coma. Chemical pneumonitis may also be a complication but tends to resolve completely and rapidly. Rarely, liver cell damage may be a feature of chlorhexidine ingestion.

Phenols are more toxic. Not uncommonly spillage on to the face and chest occurs during ingestion. Initially the lesions are white and become brown in a few days. The burns are said to be painless because of destruction of the nerve endings. Coma may supervene and hypotension, shock and hypothermia are common. A severe metabolic acidosis is usually present and laryngeal oedema, respiratory failure, myocardial damage and renal failure may develop. Aspiration into the lungs produces a haemorrhagic tracheobronchitis and pneumonitis. In rare cases methaemoglobinaemia and intravascular haemolysis have been reported. The urine is usually grey or black in colour and, together with the breath, blood and gastric contents, may smell strongly of phenol.

Management

Gastric emptying is contraindicated. Demulcents may be of symptomatic value. Upper alimentary endoscopy may be indicated if serious corrosive effects are suspected. Corticosteroids or, rarely, tracheostomy may be necessary for laryngeal oedema. Metabolic acidosis should be corrected and other supportive measures implemented according to the patient's condition. The possibility that isopropanol is contributing to the clinical picture should be considered and treated appropriately if present (p. 139).

There is extremely little objective information about the value of methods to enhance elimination of absorbed phenols. In one case haemodialysis failed to remove significant quantities of cresol. Alkalinization of the urine and plasmapheresis may be worth trying in severe DCMX intoxication since it is more soluble in alkaline than acid media and is concentrated several-fold in red blood cells.

References

Brook MP, McCarron MM, Mueller JA. Pine oil cleaner ingestion. *Ann Emerg Med* 1989; **18**: 391–395.

Roche S, Chinn R, Webb S. Chlorhexidine-induced gastritis. *Postgrad Med J* 1991; **67**: 210–211.

Shipton EA, Muller FO, Steyn EP. Dettol (chloroxylenol and terpineol) poisoning in a pregnant patient. *S Afr Med J* 1984; **66**: 822.

Ergotamine

General considerations

Poisoning with ergotamine tartrate is usually chronic or subacute and due to therapeutic overdosage with antimigraine preparations. Acute poisoning with a single large dose is rare.

Features

The features of poisoning are mainly due to diffuse, symmetrical constriction of peripheral arteries, particularly those in the legs. Paraesthesiae, numbness, pain and feelings of cold in one or more limbs result and the skin is pale or cyanosed with reduced temperature. Digital gangrene may develop in severe poisoning and in subacute cases there may be a history of intermittent claudication. Peripheral pulses may be reduced or impalpable and the blood pressure is correspondingly low. The arteries supplying internal organs are also affected and mesenteric ischaemia, myocardial infarction, stroke, and acute and chronic renal failure have all been recorded. Consciousness may be impaired after acute overdosage but in some cases this will be due to CNS depressants included in some migraine preparations. Tachycardia, hypotension, raised respiratory rate, haemorrhagic gastritis and cerebral oedema have been reported. Overdosage in late pregnancy has caused frequent uterine contractions and fetal death.

Management

Repeated doses of oral activated charcoal should be given. Analgesics may be required for severe ischaemic pain. Various measures, including vasodilators, heparin, sympathetic block and low molecular weight dextran have been used in patients with severe arterial insufficiency but their value is uncertain. Most patients improve with stopping the drug and simple symptomatic measures. Sodium nitroprusside is probably the drug of choice should a vasodilator be indicated.

References

Au KL, Woo JSK, Wong VCW. Intrauterine death from ergotamine overdosage. *Eur J Obstet Gynecol Reprod Biol* 1985; **19**: 313–315.
Deviere J, Reuse C, Askenasi R. Ischemic pancreatitis and hepatitis secondary to ergotamine poisoning. *J Clin Gastroenterol* 1987; **9**: 350–352.

Ethanol

General considerations

Ethanol (ethyl alcohol) is toxicologically important, not only as a poison in its own right, but because it is ubiquitous and potentiates the CNS depressant effects of other psychotropic drugs. For some years 60–70% of self-poisoning episodes in men and a smaller but increasing percentage of those in women have been associated with the consumption of alcohol. As a result, it is frequently difficult to assess the extent to which a patient's clinical condition is the result of ethanol and how much is due to other drugs taken simultaneously.

Chronic ingestion of excessive quantities of ethanol is also important since it induces the hepatic microsomal oxidase enzyme system, thereby allowing the alcoholic patient to metabolize some drugs more rapidly. This effect may act to advantage when barbiturates are taken in overdosage but is a disadvantage when paracetamol (acetaminophen) is taken.

Ethanol is mainly metabolized in the liver to acetaldehyde and thence to acetate. The reactions are catalysed by alcohol and aldehyde dehydrogenases. Alcohol dehydrogenase is readily saturated and ethanol is removed according to zero-order kinetics at a rate of about 10 ml/hour.

Features

Poisoning with ethanol produces varying degrees of CNS depression including coma, hypotension, hypothermia, respiratory failure and death. The breath usually has a characteristic odour and there is an ever-present risk of vomiting, aspiration into the lungs and respiratory obstruction. Arterial blood gas analysis often shows a mild metabolic acidosis. Ethanol-induced hypoglycaemia is uncommon in adults but has been reported to occur in up to 12% of children.

Management

Gastric lavage rarely retrieves significant quantities of ethanol and is only indicated in unconscious patients, provided the airway can be protected. Charcoal does not bind ethanol and is therefore of no value. Treatment is supportive and significant improvement within a few hours can be confidently expected. Head injury should be excluded. Ethanol is readily removed by haemodialysis but it is doubtful if this form of treatment should ever be necessary for uncomplicated poisoning.

Blood ethanol concentrations

Blood ethanol concentrations are most accurately measured by gas–liquid chromatography but few hospital laboratories are able to provide this analysis on an emergency basis. Breath alcohol analysers give a reasonable indication of the magnitude of the blood ethanol concentration and can be used at the bedside. On average, they decline by about 200 mg/l per hour but there is considerable interindividual variation.

Blood ethanol concentrations in poisoned patients vary widely but values up to 3 g/l are commonplace and there are reports of uneventful recovery from concentrations of 6–8 g/l.

References

Beattie JO, Hull D, Cockburn F. Children intoxicated by alcohol in Nottingham and Glasgow, 1973–84. *Br Med J* 1986; **292**: 519–521.

Gershman H, Steeper J. Rate of clearance of ethanol from the blood of intoxicated patients in the emergency department. *J Emerg Med* 1991; **9**: 307–311.

Minion GE, Slovis CM, Boutiette L. Severe alcohol intoxication: a study of 204 consecutive patients. *Clin Toxicol* 1989; **27**: 375–384.

Pollack CV, Jorden RC, Carlton FB *et al.* Gastric emptying in the acutely inebriated patient. *J Emerg Med* 1992; **10**: 1–5.

Ethylene glycol

General considerations

Ethylene glycol is readily available as the major constituent of antifreeze preparations and de-icers. It has a bitter-sweet taste and may be drunk accidentally by children or intentionally by adults, either for deliberate self-poisoning or as a substitute for alcohol. It is metabolized by alcohol dehydrogenase to glycolaldehyde and glycolic, glyoxylic and oxalic acids. The early features of toxicity are due to the substance itself but the later, more serious consequences are thought to be due to its metabolites. Glycolic acid is responsible for the severe metabolic acidosis which develops while oxalic acid combines with plasma calcium to form insoluble calcium oxalate which is deposited as crystals in the brain, heart and kidneys.

Diagnosis

Ethylene glycol ingestion carries a significant mortality but can be treated effectively provided it is diagnosed early enough. Unfortunately, diagnosis is exceedingly difficult in the absence of a clear history of ingestion and if consciousness is impaired by the time the patient presents. A high index of suspicion is required. If less than 6 hours have passed since ingestion it may be possible to demonstrate fluorescence of the urine under a Wood's (ultraviolet) lamp since some antifreezes contain fluorescein. In other cases suspicion should be aroused by the presence of an anion-gap acidosis (p. 22) and urgent measurement of the concentration of ethylene glycol in plasma should be requested. If this is not immediately available, supplementary diagnostic clues such as hypocalcaemia, oxalate crystals in the urine sediment and a high osmolal gap should be sought.

Calculation of the osmolal gap

To determine the osmolal gap one must first measure the plasma concentrations of urea, sodium and glucose and the actual osmolality. It is vital that the latter is measured by the technique utilizing depression of freezing point since other methods are invalid. The gap is the difference between the calculated osmolality of plasma and the actual osmolality. The calculated osmolality in mosmol/kg H_2O is determined from the following equation:

$$\frac{(1.86 \times [Na^+ \text{ in mmol/l}]) + [\text{urea in mmol/l}] + [\text{glucose in mmol/l}]}{0.93}$$

In normal individuals the gap is usually <10 mosmol/kg H_2O.

Features

The course of ethylene glycol poisoning can be divided into three phases which, not infrequently, merge into each other.

During the first few hours there is ataxia, slurred speech, nausea, vomiting, occasionally minor haematemesis, convulsions and drowsiness leading to coma. A variety of ocular signs may be present including nystagmus and ophthalmoplegia. The neurological features are most prominent 6–12 hours after ingestion.

The second phase (12–24 hours after ingestion) is dominated by cardiorespiratory problems, the respiratory rate usually being increased (due to the development of metabolic acidosis), tachycardia and a slight rise in blood pressure. Convulsions and cardiac dysrhythmias may be precipitated by hypocalcaemia. Cardiac failure, bronchopneumonia and cerebral oedema may be terminal events in severe cases.

The features of the final phase are due to the onset of renal tubular necrosis with bilateral renal angle and loin pain and oliguria. A diffuse myositis may also be present.

Urine examination usually reveals albuminuria, haematuria and oxalate crystals. A polymorph leucocytosis (up to $40\,000/mm^3$) is common. The plasma potassium is raised and the bicarbonate is frequently <10 mmol/l due to severe metabolic acidosis. Hypocalcaemia may be severe. Serum creatine phosphokinase activity may be raised if a myositis is present.

Cranial nerve palsies appearing 7–14 days after ingestion have been reported. The mechanism of damage is not known.

Management

Supportive measures
The stomach should be emptied if the patient presents within 2 hours of ingestion, taking appropriate steps to protect the airway. Arterial blood gas analysis and measurement of the serum calcium should be requested urgently. Metabolic acidosis should be corrected with intravenous sodium bicarbonate – very large amounts may be necessary. An adequate fluid intake should be ensured and the urine volume must be monitored carefully to detect oliguria at the earliest moment. Acute renal failure should be managed conventionally.

Calcium administration
Hypocalcaemia requires intravenous administration of calcium gluconate (10 ml of 10% solution) if convulsions or arrhythmias are present and possibly during correction of acidosis. Caution is required, however; indiscriminate calcium replacement may only contribute to the formation of calcium oxalate crystals and their deposition in tissues.

Ethanol administration
Alcohol dehydrogenase has a much greater affinity for ethanol than for ethylene glycol and the metabolism of the latter (and therefore its toxicity) is almost totally inhibited if sufficient ethanol is given. Blood ethanol concentrations of about 1 g/l are optimal but even lower concentrations considerably slow the metabolism of ethylene glycol. Ethanol should therefore be given as soon as possible.

In the early stages of intoxication it may be given orally provided vomiting or impairment of consciousness is not present. A loading dose of 0.6 g/kg body weight is recommended and is conveniently given in the form of one of the commonly available brands of whisky, gin or vodka which contain 40 g/l ethanol. A 75 kg person will therefore need about 45 g ethanol (about 100 ml of the spirits mentioned). Maintenance doses of 60–150 mg ethanol/kg per hour will then be required.

Ethanol can also be given intravenously, the loading dose for a 75 kg person by this route being 60 ml absolute ethanol in 0.5 litre isotonic dextrose over 30 min. This is followed by 12 ml absolute ethanol/ hour.

It is important to appreciate that the amount of ethanol necessary to attain required plasma concentrations will vary considerably from one individual to another, particularly if microsomal enzymes are induced and even more so if haemodialysis is used concurrently; the laboratory must be prepared to monitor plasma levels to guide therapy.

Haemodialysis
Using ethanol to inhibit metabolism of ethylene glycol totally not only prevents toxicity but effectively blocks its elimination. Fortunately, this can be surmounted by using dialysis to remove the parent substance from the body. Haemodialysis is the most efficient technique and is therefore indicated in severe poisoning and continued until concentrations of the toxin can no longer be measured. If the latter is not possible, haemodialysis should be performed for a minimum of 8 hours and repeated if metabolic acidosis recurs after stopping.

References

Malmlund H-O, Berg A, Karlman G *et al*. Considerations for the treatment of ethylene glycol poisonings based on two cases. *Clin Toxicol* 1991; **29**: 231–240.

Spillane L, Roberts JR, Meyer AE. Multiple cranial nerve deficits after ethylene glycol poisoning. *Ann Emerg Med* 1991; **20**: 208–210.

Winter ML, Ellis MD, Snodgrass WR. Urine fluorescence using a Wood's lamp to detect the antifreeze additive sodium fluorescein: a qualitative adjunctive test in suspected ethylene glycol ingestions. *Ann Emerg Med* 1990; **19**: 663–667.

Fluoride

General considerations

Hydrogen fluoride, hydrofluoric acid and its acid salts are used in industry and poisoning in this setting is usually due to skin exposure although fluorine can also be absorbed by inhalation. Sodium fluoride was formerly used as a rodenticide and insecticide but its most common use now is in the prophylaxis of dental caries. Fortunately, in this form (up to 2.2 mg sodium fluoride per tablet – the equivalent of 1 mg fluorine ion) it is relatively safe. Young children have ingested up to 176 mg without developing anything more than alimentary symptoms. Similarly, serious toxicity after ingestion of fluoride-containing tooth-pastes is improbable. It is generally held that the toxic dose of sodium fluoride is 10–20 mg/kg body weight although symptoms have occurred at lesser doses. Fluoride is a potent inhibitor of cell metabolism and chelates calcium. Intracellular calcium levels may increase as ex-tracellular ones fall precipitously, activating calcium-dependent po-tassium channels, potassium efflux from cells and potentially fatal hyperkalaemia.

Features

The immediate effects of ingestion of inorganic fluorides are nausea, hypersalivation, vomiting, abdominal pain and diarrhoea. There may be a soapy taste in the mouth. A haemorrhagic gastroenteritis ensues. Absorbed fluoride ions chelate calcium leading to tetany, hypo-calcaemic convulsions and ventricular tachycardia and fibrillation with some victims having as many as 50 or 60 episodes of fibrillation despite antidysrhythmic therapy. Hyperkalaemia may be an important contribu-tor to cardiotoxicity. Coma occurs due to hypoxia and a direct CNS effect of the fluoride. Respiratory failure and acute renal tubular necrosis may develop. Laboratory investigation confirms hypocalcae-mia and the plasma magnesium concentration may also be reduced. There is often a severe metabolic acidosis.

Inhalation of hydrogen fluoride produces laryngeal and pulmonary oedema. Fluoride skin burns are usually deep, exceedingly painful and may result in profound hypocalcaemia within 2–3 hours.

Management

Ingestion
Ingestion of more than 30 mg sodium fluoride/kg body weight should be managed by emptying the stomach and giving milk, calcium gluconate or aluminium hydroxide by mouth to bind fluoride in the gut. The cardiac rhythm must be monitored continuously and facilities for defibrillation and assisted respiration should be immediately available. Acid–base disturbances, hypocalcaemia and hyperkalaemia should be sought and corrected. Very large quantities of calcium gluconate may be necessary. Frequent measurement of the serum calcium is essential and a good urinary output will promote fluoride excretion. Haemodialysis has occasionally been used to eliminate inorganic fluoride but should rarely be required.

Ingestion of less than 10 mg sodium fluoride/kg body weight does not require admission to hospital or treatment other than liberal quantities of milk, while children who have taken intermediate doses (10–30 mg/kg) should be managed similarly but observed for a few hours.

Fluoride burns
Injection of calcium gluconate around fluoride skin burns and application of calcium gluconate gel to the damaged surface reduce the risk of systemic fluoride intoxication but surgical advice about management of the skin ulcers will be required. Systemic features should be managed as above.

References

Augenstein WL, Spoerke DG, Kulig KW *et al*. Fluoride ingestion in children: a review of 87 cases. *Pediatrics* 1991; **88**: 907–912.
Bayless JM, Tinanoff N. Diagnosis and treatment of acute fluoride toxicity. *J Am Dent Assoc* 1985; **110**: 209–211.
Bertolini JC. Hydrofluoric acid: a review of toxicity. *J Emerg Med* 1992; **10**: 163–168.

Fluoxetine and fluvoxamine

General considerations

Fluoxetine is a new antidepressant and, like zimeldine (now no longer marketed) and fluvoxamine, is a serotonin uptake inhibitor which does not have the anticholinergic actions of the tricyclic antidepressants. Experience of overdosage with it is limited but it seems that doses of up to 3.6 mg/kg body weight do not cause symptoms. Larger amounts are also relatively safe unless potentiated by ethanol. There is even less information on overdosage with fluvoxamine and most of the cases reported cannot be interpreted because of simultaneous ingestion of other drugs. It is said to have a mean plasma half-life of 15 hours.

Features

Most patients will have no features of toxicity. Drowsiness and sinus tachycardia are the most common effects but nausea and diarrhoea have also been reported. Junctional bradycardia, seizures and hypertension have been encountered rarely and flu-like symptoms may develop after a day or two. Until more information is forthcoming, the features of fluvoxamine overdosage should be considered similar to those of fluoxetine.

Management

Supportive and symptomatic measures are all that are required. Activated charcoal should be given.

Reference

Borys DJ, Setzer SC, Ling LJ *et al*. The effects of fluoxetine in the overdose patient. *Clin Toxicol* 1990; **28**: 331–340.

Gamma-hexachlorocyclohexane

General considerations

Gamma-hexachlorocyclohexane (otherwise known as gamma-HCH, gamma-benzene hexachloride or lindane) is an insecticide widely used in agriculture and as a 1% solution for the treatment of scabies and pediculosis. It is readily and rapidly absorbed through the gastrointestinal tract and skin and is highly lipid-soluble. Acute poisoning is uncommon but more frequent in children.

Features

Consciousness is rapidly lost and myoclonus may occur. Muscle tone is greatly increased and the reflexes are exaggerated. Vomiting is common and constantly threatens the airway. Convulsions are the major feature of acute intoxication and rhabdomyolysis, severe acidosis and disseminated intravascular coagulation may ensue. Renal tubular and hepatocellular necrosis, pancreatitis and proximal myopathy with myoglobinuria have been reported as delayed complications.

A polymorph leucocytosis is commonly found and serum aspartate aminotransferase and lactic dehydrogenase activity may be increased.

Management

There is no specific treatment for this type of poisoning. The stomach should be emptied if the poison has been taken within 4 hours and after taking appropriate steps to safeguard the airway. Arterial blood gas analysis should be carried out and any acid–base abnormality corrected. The combination of coma, vomiting and convulsions is particularly dangerous. Isolated convulsions do not require treatment but if frequent, control is best obtained by curarization and mechanical ventilation rather than with intravenous diazepam alone. Other problems are treated symptomatically as they arise.

Prognosis

Gamma-HCH is rapidly metabolized and redistributed in adipose tissue. Recovery of consciousness can be expected within about 12 hours. Convulsions subside during this time but the patient may remain drowsy and irritable for 24–48 hours. Once consciousness is regained survival is likely.

References

Kurt TL, Best R, Read G *et al*. Accidental Kwell (lindane) ingestion. *Vet Hum Toxicol* 1986; **28**: 569–571.
Sunder Ram Rao CV, Shreenivas R, Singh V *et al*. Disseminated intravascular coagulation in a case of fatal lindane poisoning. *Vet Hum Toxicol* 1988; **30**: 132–134.

H₁-receptor antihistamines

Astemizole   Terfenadine

General considerations

Although these newer antihistamines are being increasingly used, information on the effects of overdosage with them is still limited. They are subject to extensive first-pass metabolism.

Features

H_1-receptor antagonists appear to lack the anticholinergic actions of older antihistamines. Nothing more than drowsiness developed in a 14-year-old girl who ingested 200 mg astemizole but the QT_c interval was prolonged in younger children who were thought to have taken 2.5–16.7 mg/kg body weight. Ventricular tachycardia has been reported in children and adults. In some cases it was of the torsade de pointes type or with associated giant U waves.

It is thought that up to 120 mg terfenadine will not produce toxicity in young children but they did not have electrocardiograms to exclude subclinical cardiotoxicity. Prolongation of the QT_c interval, ventricular dysrhythmias and convulsions has been produced by larger amounts in adults.

Management

Until the toxicity of these compounds in overdose is more clearly defined, it would seem wise to observe these patients for a minimum of

12 hours. An electrocardiogram should be carried out and the heart monitored if the QT interval is prolonged. Only a small minority will require active measures. Oral activated charcoal may be given but it did not prevent cardiotoxicity in some children. Complications are managed as they arise. Intravenous magnesium sulphate appeared to abolish ventricular ectopic beats and tachycardia in one man.

References

Hoppu K, Tikanoja T, Tapanainen P et al. Accidental astemizole overdose in young children. Lancet 1991; **338**: 538–540.

Leor J, Harman M, Rabinowitz B et al. Giant U waves and associated ventricular tachycardia complicating astemizole overdose: successful therapy with intravenous magnesium. Am J Med 1991; **91**: 94–97.

Spiller HA, Picciotti M, Perez E. Accidental terfenadine ingestion in children. Vet Hum Toxicol 1989; **31**: 154–156.

H_2-receptor antihistamines

Chlorpheniramine   Promethazine
Diphenhydramine   Trimeprazine
Methapyrilene

General considerations

These older antihistamines are still widely used for control of allergic conditions and in some pleasantly flavoured cough mixtures. They have sedative and marked anticholinergic actions. Overdosage with them is not uncommon but is rarely serious and they are also taken for 'kicks'. Poisoning may also result from percutaneous absorption of anti-histamine-containing creams.

Features

The features of overdosage with this group of compounds are similar to those caused by tricyclic antidepressants (see p. 66) but the more serious complications of the latter (such as convulsions, coma and cardiac dysrhythmias) are much less common.

Management

Management is as for amitriptyline (p. 68).

References

Farrell M, Heinrichs M, Tilbelli JA. Response of life threatening dimenhydrinate intoxication to sodium bicarbonate. *Clin Toxicol* 1991; **29**: 527–535.

Köppel C, Tenczer J. Poisoning with over-the-counter doxylamine preparations: an evaluation of 109 cases. *Hum Toxicol* 1987; **6**: 355–359.

Rinder CS, Amato D, Rinder HM *et al.* Survival in complicated diphenhydramine overdose. *Crit Care Med* 1988; **16**: 1161–1162.

Schreiber W, Pauls AM, Krieg J-C. Toxische Psychose als Akutmanifestation der Diphenhydraminvergiftung. *Dtsch Med Wochenschr* 1988; **113**: 180–183.

Woodward GA, Baldassano RN. Topical diphenhydramine toxicity in a five year old with varicella. *Pediatr Emerg Care* 1988; **4**: 18–20.

Young GB, Boyd D, Kreeft J. Dimenhydrinate: evidence for dependence and tolerance. *CMAJ* 1988; **138**: 437–438.

Holly

General considerations

The attractive red berries of the holly tree, *Ilex aquifolium*, appear around Christmas and are commonly eaten by children. They contain ilexanthin and ilex acid.

Features

Even after eating up to 20 berries the majority of children suffer no ill effects. A few may develop vomiting, abdominal pain and diarrhoea.

Management

Treatment is usually superfluous. Symptomatic measures may be necessary in a small proportion of cases.

Honeysuckle

General considerations

The berries of honeysuckle (*Lonicera* species) are occasionally eaten by children. They contain cyanogenic glycosides, alkaloids and saponins. The latter are probably responsible for clinical toxicity.

Features

The majority of children suffer no ill effects but a few develop vomiting and abdominal pain.

Management

Treatment is usually superfluous. Symptomatic measures may be necessary in a small proportion of cases.

Household products

General considerations

Numerous chemical-containing products are kept in homes and contribute to ease of upkeep and the quality of life in general. However, they tend to be ingested in varying amounts by young children. Main groups of household products are considered separately, including bleaches (p. 84), corrosive agents (p. 106), disc batteries (p. 77), disinfectants (p. 116), polishes and paraffin (p. 191) and soaps, detergents and fabric conditioners (p. 213).

Features

In general, childhood exposure to household products causes very few, if any, symptoms or signs and the reader should consult sections on specific agents for those which develop in rare cases.

Ingestion of 40 match heads containing potassium bichromate has been reported to cause acute renal failure in a child while sodium dichloroisocyanurate-containing sterilizing tablets cause upper alimentary and respiratory tract corrosive lesions. Essential plant oils such as camphor, clove oil (applied locally for relief of dental pain) and others in inhalant capsules and oral preparations for use in chronic respiratory disease (Karvol and olbas oil) are potentially neurotoxic in relatively small amounts.

Ingestion of naphthalene by children who suffer from glucose-6-phosphate dehydrogenase deficiency has caused severe haemolytic anaemia.

Exposure to 'superglues' sticks digits, lips or eyelids together and generates considerable alarm. Involvement of eyes may lead to corneal damage.

Management

Management should be appropriate to the expected toxicity of the product and, in general, will be symptomatic and supportive.

Superglue exposures should be managed as follows:

1 The bonded surfaces (where practicable) should be immersed in warm water and the edges rolled against each other or separation with a blunt object attempted. Do not try to pull or cut them apart.

2 Solvents such as toluene and xylene may be helpful but are toxic and must be used sparingly and cautiously.

3 If measures 1 and 2 are unsuccessful and the affected parts are not vital, time should be allowed to pass until natural desquamation of the underlying epithelium makes separation easier.

4 Contaminated eyes must be irrigated immediately (p. 109) and assessed in the usual way, particularly to rule out mechanical injury.

References

Dean B, Krenzelok EP. Cyanoacrylates and corneal abrasion. *Clin Toxicol* 1989; **27**: 169–172.

Lane BW, Ellenhorn MJ, Hulbert TV *et al*. Clove oil ingestion in an infant. *Hum Exp Toxicol* 1991; **10**: 291–294.

Siodlak MZ, Gleeson MJ, Wengraf CL. Accidental ingestion of sterilising tablets by children. *Br Med J* 1985; **290**: 1707–1708.

Todisco V, Lamour J, Finberg L. Hemolysis from exposure to naphthalene mothballs. *N Engl J Med* 1991; **325**: 1660.

Williams DC. Acute respiratory obstruction caused by ingestion of a caustic substance. *Br Med J* 1985; **291**: 313–314.

Ibuprofen

General considerations

Ibuprofen, one of the most widely used non-steroidal anti-inflammatory drugs, is a propionic acid derivative and is available over the counter in many countries. It is rapidly absorbed from the gut, extensively metabolized and eliminated with a plasma half-life of about 3 hours after overdosage.

Features

Ibuprofen is generally of low toxicity after overdosage but a small number of cases with life-threatening and fatal consequences have been reported. In large series only about 20% of patients developed symptoms. Ingestion of less than 100 mg/kg body weight is unlikely to cause features in a child while more than 400 mg/kg may cause serious toxicity. Features are highly unlikely to develop for the first time later than 4 hours after the overdose was taken.

Drowsiness, vomiting, abdominal discomfort, tinnitus, blurred vision and tachycardia are the most common features. The more serious include coma, convulsions, apnoea and bradycardia. Liver and renal function tests may become abnormal and acute renal failure has been described very rarely.

Management

Patients who have ingested less than 100 mg ibuprofen/kg body weight do not require treatment nor do those who are asymptomatic 4 or more hours after ingestion. Those who have taken larger amounts should receive activated charcoal. Treatment thereafter is supportive, the airway and ventilation being maintained as necessary. The plasma half-life of ibuprofen is so short that elimination techniques are irrelevant.

References

Hall AH, Smolinske SC, Stover B *et al*. Ibuprofen overdose in adults. *Clin Toxicol* 1992; **30**: 23–37.

Menzies DG, Conn AG, Williamson IJ *et al*. Fulminant hyperkalaemia and multiple complications following ibuprofen overdose. *Med Toxicol Adverse Drug Exp* 1989; **4**: 468–471.

Perazella MA, Buller GK. Can ibuprofen cause acute renal failure in a normal individual? A case of acute overdose. *Am J Kidney Dis* 1991; **18**: 600–602.

Insulin

General considerations

Most individuals who deliberately inject themselves with large doses of insulin are insulin-dependent diabetics though occasionally their non-diabetic relatives, and doctors or nurses, may do so. The incidence of self-poisoning with insulin may be higher than the relatively small number of cases reported in the literature would suggest. Virtually every type of insulin has been used for self-poisoning and occasionally for murder.

Features

The patient may be a known diabetic or have evidence of repeated injection over the thighs. It is not uncommon to find an empty syringe and vials by the patient. Examination will reveal the usual signs of hypoglycaemia and the diagnosis may be rapidly confirmed by measurement of the blood glucose concentration and by the clinical response to intravenous glucose. Cerebral oedema and brain damage may occur if hypoglycaemia is severe and protracted before treatment is started.

Frequently the severity of hypoglycaemia is not as marked as might be anticipated from the quantity of insulin injected, suggesting that there is a system which limits the blood glucose response to plasma insulin and is not affected by major increases in circulating insulin levels. The limited severity of hypoglycaemia after overdosage in some cases may be one of the factors leading to underdetection of this type of self-poisoning.

Management

If there is any clinical suspicion of hypoglycaemia, whether or not due to insulin overdosage, the blood glucose should be measured to substantiate the diagnosis and 50 ml of 50% glucose injected intravenously. Occasionally this dose will have to be repeated before a response is obtained. It is then advisable to give a constant infusion of 10% dextrose. Additional boluses of glucose may be required should hypoglycaemia recur. Hypokalaemia must be corrected. The patient should also be given a carbohydrate-rich meal as soon as he or she is able to eat. Cerebral oedema should be treated conventionally (p. 53).

Prognosis

The majority of patients make a complete recovery though there is a risk of recurrent hypoglycaemia depending upon the duration of action of the insulin involved. There is no evidence that acute massive overdosage alters future long-term insulin requirements.

Plasma insulin concentrations

Plasma insulin concentrations correlate well with the quantities stated to have been injected and immunoreactive insulin levels of up to 32 000 mu/ml have been found after self-poisoning.

References

Kaminer Y, Robbins DR. Attempted suicide by insulin overdose in insulin-dependent diabetic adolescents. *Pediatrics* 1988; **81**: 526–528.
Samuels MH, Eckel RH. Massive insulin overdose: detailed studies of free insulin levels and glucose requirements. *J Toxicol Clin Toxicol* 1989; **27**: 157–168.

Iron

General considerations

Although acute iron poisoning has been a problem for many years, there is still much to learn about its pathophysiology and management. It is predominantly a childhood problem though adults occasionally ingest large quantities in self-poisoning episodes. There are numerous iron preparations on the market and their widespread prescription for anaemia, presumed anaemia and during pregnancy makes them readily available to all age groups including young children. Moreover, the

Table 4.2 The elemental iron content of commonly used preparations

Product	Amount/tablet (mg)	Elemental iron (mg)
Ferrous fumarate	200	65
Ferrous gluconate	300	35
Ferrous glycine sulphate	225	40
Ferrous succinate	100	35
Ferrous sulphate	200	60
Ferrous sulphate (dried)	200	60

brightly coloured tablets may be indistinguishable from sweets. The incidence of this common and particularly serious childhood poisoning could be reduced by better care of medicines in the home and insistence on iron tablets being dispensed in child-resistant containers.

A distinction must be drawn between the amount of an iron salt in a tablet or syrup and its elemental iron content. The latter is the important toxicological consideration and the elemental iron content of some common iron preparations is given in Table 4.2. The fatal amount of elemental iron is estimated to be between 180 and 300 mg/kg body weight.

Features

General
Serious toxicity is unlikely unless >60 mg elemental iron/kg body weight has been ingested.

The clinical course of acute iron poisoning is traditionally divided into four phases. The first comprises the first few hours after ingestion when vomiting, diarrhoea and abdominal pain are common. The vomitus and stools are usually dark grey or black due to the disintegrating iron preparation but may later become blood-stained due to corrosive effects on the upper gastrointestinal mucosa. The majority of mild poisonings do not progress beyond this point and symptoms settle within 6–8 hours. In severe poisoning first-phase features also include drowsiness, coma, convulsions, metabolic acidosis and shock (which is often more severe than would be expected from the amount of gastrointestinal fluid and blood loss). It has been attributed to the effect of circulating free iron (i.e. serum iron in excess of the expected total iron-binding capacity) and release of vasodilator material from the liver. A few patients die in this phase from progressive circulatory failure and coma.

During the second phase, starting 6–12 hours after ingestion, symptoms abate as the iron is taken up by the reticuloendothelial system. After a lull of 12–48 hours a minority of patients enter the third phase in which there is severe shock, metabolic acidosis, jaundice with its attendant coagulation abnormalities, hypoglycaemia and renal failure. Intestinal infarction has also been reported. The mortality in this phase is high and the liver usually shows hepatocellular necrosis most marked in the periportal regions. Rarely, infection with *Yersinia enterocolitica* may develop 2–3 days after the overdose.

The final phase of iron poisoning is due to gastric stricture formation and pyloric stenosis (alone or in combination) with obstructive symptoms starting after 2–5 weeks.

Serum iron concentrations and assessment of severity of poisoning

Although a straight abdominal X-ray may help substantiate the approximate number of tablets ingested it is customary to assess the severity of poisoning by measuring the serum iron concentration as an emergency. The total iron-binding capacity may be falsely raised and is of no value. Initial serum iron concentrations in poisoned children have been correlated with the presence of shock and/or coma, the generally accepted clinical indices of severe poisoning. On the basis of these data it has been recommended that an initial serum iron concentration greater than 5000 µg/l (90 µmol/l) is an indication for energetic treatment with chelating agents. However, several reservations must be noted.

1 The kinetics of iron after acute overdosage in humans have not been adequately investigated but serum concentrations probably peak within 4 hours and fall rapidly thereafter. It follows that the time interval influences the level above which treatment may be necessary. It is thus inappropriate to recommend that a single iron concentration should be an indication for treatment.
2 Interpretation of serum iron levels will be even more difficult when slow-release formulations have been ingested, though there is as yet no published evidence on this point.
3 Concern has been expressed about hypotension, anaphylaxis and rashes from desferrioxamine and it is desirable to avoid unnecessary treatment. In one study, over 60% of children with initial serum iron concentrations above 5000 µg/l (90 µmol/l) did not have clinically severe poisoning.

The decision to treat iron poisoning with desferrioxamine requires thought and judgment rather than slavish obedience to an arbitrary iron concentration.

Management

Referral to hospital

Patients who have taken <20 mg iron/kg do not require treatment or referral to hospital. Ingestion of 20–60 mg/kg is an indication for gastric emptying but admission to hospital is probably unnecessary unless symptoms are present. Those who have ingested larger quantities require admission.

Preventing absorption

The stomach should be emptied if >20 mg elemental iron/kg body weight has been ingested within 4 hours.

Various lavage fluids and additives to them have been recommended on the basis that their use would reduce absorption even further than could be achieved by water alone. They include adding desferrioxamine (2 g powder/l of water) to the lavage fluid to chelate iron remaining in the stomach and leaving a further 10 g in the stomach at the end of the procedure – an expensive measure. This is not recommended; it may not prevent absorption of the amounts of iron commonly involved in poisoning episodes and the absorbed iron–desferrioxamine complex (ferrioxamine) may cause serious hypotension. Sodium bicarbonate and disodium phosphate solutions complex with iron to form the relatively insoluble carbonates and phosphates respectively. However, there is no evidence that they are of clinical value and disodium phosphate may produce life-threatening hypocalcaemia and hyperphosphataemia.

If a slow-release iron formulation has been ingested and tablets remain in the bowel after gastric lavage the use of whole-bowel irrigation (p. 42) is probably more useful.

Supportive measures

Arterial blood gas analysis is mandatory in severe iron poisoning and any acid–base disturbance should be corrected. Liver function tests, particularly the prothrombin time, must be monitored at least daily if severe liver damage is suspected. Adequate replacement of fluid and blood losses is essential. Hepatic and renal failure should be managed conventionally.

Desferrioxamine

Parenteral desferrioxamine is the treatment of choice for severe iron poisoning. It should be given immediately, without waiting for the serum iron concentration, if it is clinically obvious that poisoning is severe (i.e. coma or shock are present). It is usually given intra-muscularly (2 g for an adult and 1 g for a child) combined with intravenous infusion at a rate which must not exceed 15 mg/kg per hour to avoid hypotension. The total intravenous dose should not exceed 80 mg/kg in 24 hours. The iron–desferrioxamine complex is excreted in the urine, making it orange-red in colour, and may be eliminated by dialysis if renal failure develops. Administration of the antidote may be stopped when the patient is clinically improved, free iron is no longer present in the plasma or the urinary screen for iron is negative.

Poisoning in pregnancy
Acute iron overdosage in pregnancy is not uncommon and may be fatal for the mother and fetus. It must be managed as occurring in other situations. Concern over possible teratogenic effects of desferrioxamine is not a reason for withholding the antidote.

Prognosis

Previous estimates indicating a high mortality from acute iron poisoning were almost certainly biased by the tendency to report only severe and fatal cases. The overall mortality is probably much less than 5% but survival from serious poisoning depends upon administration of desferrioxamine at the earliest possible moment.

References

Everson GW, Bertaccini EJ, O'Leary J *et al.* Use of whole bowel irrigation in an infant following an iron overdose. *Am J Emerg Med* 1991; **9**: 366–369.

Klein-Schwartz W, Oderda GM, Gorman RL *et al.* Assessment of management guidelines. Acute iron ingestion. *Clin Pediatr* 1990; **29**: 316–321.

McElhatton PR, Roberts JC, Sullivan FM. The consequences of iron overdose and its treatment in pregnancy. *Hum Exp Toxicol* 1991; **10**: 251–259.

Milteer RM, Sarpong S, Poydras U. *Yersinia enterocolitica* septicemia after accidental iron overdose. *Pediatr Infect Dis J* 1989; **8**: 537–538.

Schauben JL, Augenstein L, Cox J *et al.* Iron poisoning: report of three cases and a review of therapeutic intervention. *J Emerg Med* 1990; **8**: 309–319.

Tenenbein M. The total iron-binding capacity in iron poisoning. *AJDC* 1991; **145**: 437–439.

Tenenbein M, Kopelow ML, deSa DJ. Myocardial failure and shock in iron poisoning. *Hum Toxicol* 1988; **7**: 281–284.

Tenenbein M, Littman C, Stimpson RE. Gastrointestinal pathology in adult iron overdose. *Clin Toxicol* 1990; **28**: 311–320.

Isoniazid

General considerations

Acute isoniazid overdosage is uncommon. Though most cases are the result of deliberate self-poisoning it has been suggested that others may be attempts to obtain an LSD-type 'trip'. Ingestion of 1.5 g by an adult would be expected to cause minor toxicity while more than 15 g is potentially fatal.

Isoniazid is acetylated in the liver and individuals may be 'slow' or 'fast' acetylators, the proportion of each varying from one society to another and being genetically determined. The significance of this after massive overdosage has not been investigated. Very little isoniazid is excreted unchanged in the urine.

Isoniazid toxicity is thought to be due to acute pyridoxine (vitamin B_6) deficiency and reduction in brain gamma-aminobutyric acid, the transmitter which inhibits convulsions.

Features

Symptoms usually develop within 2–4 hours. In the early stages nausea, vomiting, hallucinations and visions of brightly coloured lights have been described but approximately half the patients develop some impairment of consciousness and about 90% have one or more convulsions. Consciousness may not be regained between seizures and the patient may remain cyanosed with a tachycardia. There is an ever-present risk of aspiration of gastric contents and respiratory failure. A severe metabolic acidosis is common and is due to raised serum lactate concentrations secondary to hypoxia and convulsions. Hyperpyrexia, rhabdomyolysis and acute renal failure may also develop.

Hyperglycaemia and a polymorph leucocytosis occur frequently and elevation of serum osmolality, aspartate aminotransferase and lactate dehydrogenase has been noted occasionally. Transient peripheral neuropathy was described in one man treated by haemodialysis.

Management

The first priorities are to establish and maintain a patent airway and to control convulsions. The latter may be refractory to conventional measures until large quantities of pyridoxine have been given. The dose for an adult is 1 g intravenously for each gram of isoniazid ingested or, if the latter is unknown, 5 g in 50 ml intravenously over 5 min and repeated at intervals of 20–30 min until convulsions cease and consciousness is regained. Once the patient's condition has stabilized repeated oral charcoal should be given if the airway can be protected. Metabolic acidosis and hypoxia are first corrected by controlling convulsions but intravenous sodium bicarbonate may be necessary.

Attempts to enhance the elimination of isoniazid are usually superfluous. Forced diuresis would not be expected to be beneficial since little drug is excreted unchanged. Haemodialysis and charcoal haemoperfusion have been recommended but should not be necessary except in very severe intoxication. Plasma isoniazid concentrations rarely exceed 150 mg/l although values up to 250 mg/l 6 hours after ingestion have been reported.

References

Bredemann JA, Krechel SW, Eggers GWN. Treatment of refractory seizures in massive isoniazid overdose. *Anesth Analg* 1990; **71**: 554–557.

Orlowski JP, Paganini EP, Pippenger CE. Treatment of a potentially lethal dose isoniazid ingestion. *Ann Emerg Med* 1988; **17**: 73–76.

Siefkin AD, Albertson TE, Corbett MG. Isoniazid overdose: pharmacokinetics and effects of oral charcoal in treatment. *Hum Toxicol* 1987; **6**: 497–501.

Isopropanol

General considerations

Isopropanol (isopropyl alcohol) is a constituent of a variety of preparations including disinfectants, solvents, windscreen washes, cosmetics and pharmaceutical preparations. In some countries it is available in a 70% solution as a 'rubbing alcohol'. Percutaneous absorption is low but poisoning can readily occur by inhalation. Usually, however, it is the result of ingestion, often by alcoholics seeking a substitute for ethanol. One case of rectal self-administration has been described. Isopropanol is metabolized by alcohol dehydrogenase, the principal metabolite being acetone.

Features

The features of isopropanol intoxication resemble those of ethanol poisoning with loss of consciousness, vasodilatation, hypotension, respiratory depression, hyporeflexia and hypothermia. However, the characteristic odour of ethanol on the breath is absent. Patients who become severely hypotensive usually die. The CNS depressant effect of isopropanol is twice that of the same volume of ethanol. Nausea, vomiting and abdominal pain are commoner than with ethanol and a haemorrhagic gastritis may occur. Renal failure, rhabdomyolysis, myoglobinuria, haemolytic anaemia and elevation of the cerebrospinal fluid protein content are rare complications.

Acetone may be detected in the breath, blood and urine.

Management

The vast majority of patients require no more than gastric emptying and supportive measures. Haemodialysis readily removes isopropanol and its metabolites and its use should be considered in patients who are desperately ill (see the criteria for haemoperfusion, p. 51) and have high plasma isopropanol concentrations (usually greater than 4 g/l).

Plasma isopropanol concentrations

Plasma concentrations up to 5.8 g/l have been reported in severely poisoned patients. The plasma half-life of isopropanol varies from 3 to 16 hours and that for acetone from 7 to 26 hours.

References

Pappas AA, Ackerman BH, Olsen KM *et al*. Isopropanol ingestion: a report of six episodes with isopropanol and acetone serum concentration time data. *Clin Toxicol* 1991; **29**: 11–21.

Rich J, Scheife RT, Katz N *et al*. Isopropyl alcohol intoxication. *Arch Neurol* 1990; **47**: 322–324.

Laburnum

General considerations

In the UK laburnum (*Laburnum anagroides*) is probably the most common plant poison encountered in clinical practice. The laburnum tree flowers in the late spring and early summer and for some months bears pods resembling small peas containing up to eight seeds. All parts of the plant, particularly the bark and seeds, are poisonous and it is usually the latter that are involved in childhood poisoning. Cytosine, an alkaloid, is the major toxic agent.

Features

The vast majority of children do not eat enough laburnum seeds to develop symptoms. In rare cases, nausea, vomiting, hypersalivation, drowsiness, incoordination, muscle twitching and convulsions occur. Mydriasis and a tachycardia may be present. Only one death from laburnum poisoning has been recorded in the UK in the last 50 years.

Management

Treatment is usually superfluous. It has been suggested that the stomach should be emptied but even this is debatable unless a large number of seeds has been ingested. Routine hospitalization is unnecessary and it is sufficient to inform parents about the symptoms that can occur and to advise them to bring the child back to hospital should they develop. In these cases supportive care is all that can be offered.

Reference

Forrester RM. Have you eaten laburnum? *Lancet* 1979; **i**: 1073.

Lithium

General considerations

The increasing use of lithium salts for the long-term control of manic depressive psychosis has been associated with a rise in the number of serious lithium intoxications. Most are the result of therapeutic overdosage rather than deliberate self-poisoning and occur because the margin between therapeutic and toxic doses is very small. Serum concentrations must be monitored regularly during treatment if toxicity is to be avoided. Acute overdosage in persons both on and not on lithium therapy is not uncommon.

Lithium is an alkali metal which is distributed throughout the body water and concentrated in cells although distribution from the extracellular to the intracellular compartment is relatively slow. Therapeutic use of lithium may cause thirst or polyuria (independently), renal impairment and (in about 12% of cases) nephrogenic diabetes insipidus. Since lithium is excreted entirely through the kidneys, patients on long-term treatment are particularly vulnerable to reduction in fluid intake (e.g. as a result of intercurrent physical or mental illness or additional psychotropic medication) or increased fluid loss (e.g. fever, diarrhoea, diuretic therapy or the development of diabetes insipidus), either of which may precipitate serious lithium intoxication.

Features

The early features of poisoning are nausea, vomiting and diarrhoea. The later major effects are on the brain and neuromuscular system with ataxia, coarse tremor and drowsiness progressing to coma in severe cases. Initially, muscle tone is greatly increased, cog-wheel rigidity may be present and fasciculation and myoclonus are common. The reflexes are correspondingly increased and convulsions may occur. The limbs are often held in hyperextension with an expressionless face and open eyes (so-called 'coma vigile'). Rare complications have included acute renal failure, acute diabetes insipidus, myocardial infarction and polyneuropathy.

Hypernatraemia and hypokalaemia may be found and the electrocardiogram frequently shows non-specific ST depression and T wave inversion but atrioventricular and intraventricular conduction are usually unaffected.

Serum lithium concentrations and assessment of the severity of poisoning

Serum lithium concentrations are measured by flame photometry and therapeutic concentrations lie between 0.8 and 1.2 mmol/l. In general, serum concentrations correlate poorly with the clinical severity of lithium poisoning. Serious toxicity has been reported with 'therapeutic' or only slightly elevated levels while those with acute overdosage (whether or not imposed on long-term treatment) may have no features with levels as high as 4.0 mmol/l. The combination of high concentrations and minimal toxicity after acute overdosage may be partly explained by slow distribution of the drug to the tissues in the time available since ingestion. In these cases, toxic features may appear as serum concentrations are falling. Clinical features are therefore more important than lithium levels in assessing the severity of poisoning but asymptomatic patients with high levels cannot be dismissed; toxicity is sure to develop if high concentrations persist for a few days.

Management

Supportive
If a large overdose has been taken the stomach should be emptied. Many therapeutic lithium formulations are of the sustained release variety and volunteer studies suggest that whole-bowel irrigation (p. 42) should minimize absorption. Patients who are unconscious require supportive measures but increased muscle tone, convulsions and tenacious bronchial secretions may make adequate airway care extremely difficult. Dantrolene may have a role in these cases. Intravenous fluids are essential to maintain a good urinary output and the nature of the fluids should be determined by the results of urgent measurement of the plasma urea, electrolytes and osmolality. Underlying diabetes insipidus should be strongly suspected if hypernatraemia is present at the outset and in such cases only isotonic dextrose should be given till the plasma sodium and osmolality return to normal. There is a particular risk of hypernatraemia from saline infusions in lithium poisoning. Potassium supplements should be given as required.

Enhancing elimination
Forced diuresis, peritoneal dialysis and haemodialysis have been used in attempts to eliminate circulating lithium but none is entirely satisfactory. The former carries the risk of salt and water overload and is inappropriate when renal function is impaired. It is best reserved for minor poisoning. However, one report found that the addition of low-dose dopamine (2 µg/kg per min) to saline infusion significantly increased renal lithium clearance but further studies are required to assess its therapeutic value. Clearance of lithium by peritoneal dialysis is no greater than by forced diuresis and it is of little value. Haemodialysis is the most efficient method of removing lithium from the intravascular compartment but rebound increase in serum

concentrations (up to 100%) can be expected within a few hours as the plasma re-equilibrates with the intracellular fluid. Haemodialysis must therefore be repeated frequently, allowing serum lithium concentrations to rise between dialyses.

Prognosis

Recovery from lithium poisoning may take several days because of the slow rate at which lithium can be removed from cells, particularly in the brain. Some patients die from the complications of prolonged coma despite serum lithium concentrations having fallen satisfactorily. The overall mortality in published cases is about 12%.

Survivors may be left with permanent ataxia and choreoathetosis due to damage to the basal ganglia and cerebellar connections. Nephrogenic diabetes insipidus usually disappears within a few months of stopping lithium treatment but may be permanent in some cases, thus creating problems for the future management of their psychiatric illness.

References

Chang Y-C, Yip P-K, Chiu Y-N *et al.* Severe generalized neuropathy in lithium intoxication. *Eur Neurol* 1988; **28**: 39–41.

Dyson EH, Simpson D, Prescott LF *et al.* Self-poisoning and therapeutic intoxication with lithium. *Hum Toxicol* 1987; **6**: 325–329.

Friedberg RC, Spyker DA, Herold DA. Massive overdoses with sustained-release lithium carbonate preparations: pharmacokinetic model based on two case studies. *Clin Chem* 1991; **37**: 1205–1209.

Groleau G, Barish R, Tso E *et al.* Lithium intoxication. *Am J Emerg Med* 1987; **5**: 527–532.

Macdonald TM, Cotton M, Prescott LF. Low dose dopamine in lithium poisoning. *Br J Clin Pharmacol* 1988; **26**: 195.

Perrier A, Martin P-Y, Favre H *et al.* Very severe self-poisoning lithium carbonate intoxication causing a myocardial infarction. *Chest* 1991; **100**: 863–865.

Smith SW, Ling LJ, Halstenson CE. Whole-bowel irrigation as a treatment for acute lithium overdose. *Ann Emerg Med* 1991; **20**: 536–539.

Lupin

General considerations

Lupins (*Lupinus* species) are widely cultivated as garden plants although in some countries there are wild varieties. Their toxicity varies from year to year depending on the conditions of cultivation and some non-poisonous types are used for food. However all parts of the plant, particularly the seeds, may contain toxic alkaloids (mainly of the quinolizidine group) which are not altered by drying.

Lupin seeds are most likely to be ingested by small children.

Features

It is uncommon for enough seeds to be eaten to cause symptoms but large numbers rarely cause convulsions, respiratory depression, muscular weakness and bradycardia. On the other hand, short-lived anticholinergic features have been reported.

Management

Most cases will not require treatment. The stomach should be emptied if large numbers of seeds (>25) have been ingested. Treatment thereafter is symptomatic. Activated charcoal may be of value.

Reference

Marquez RL, Gutierrez-Rave M, Miranda FI. Acute poisoning by lupin seed debittering water. *Vet Hum Toxicol* 1991; **33**: 265–267.

Lysergic acid diethylamide (LSD)

General considerations

Hospital admissions following acute intoxication with LSD are uncommon. LSD is usually taken by mouth but is occasionally dissolved and snorted for a faster effect. Its mode of action is poorly understood, but the pleasurable effects it produces are well-known. Hospital referral usually results from an acute panic reaction, a schizophrenic-like psychotic state, aggressive outbursts or, rarely, attempts at suicide or homicide.

Features

The features are usually the result of adverse reactions to 'normal' doses. The individual may be found wandering in a confused, agitated state and usually has visual hallucinations. Some patients may be wildly excited and unmanageable. Dilatation of the pupils and mild hypertension are common and occasionally body temperature is raised.

Only a few cases of massive LSD overdosage have been reported. Coma, respiratory arrest and metabolic acidosis are the dominant features. Platelet dysfunction may cause a mild generalized bleeding · tendency and polymorph leucocytosis is common.

Management

Most patients only require reassurance and sedation. One dose of chlorpromazine (50–100 mg intramuscularly) is usually adequate and preferable to diazepam. If the individual is unconscious the usual supportive measures should be taken.

Prognosis

Recovery is usually complete within a few hours although in some cases hallucinations may persist up to 48 hours and the psychotic state for 3–4 days. Even patients who had serious physical consequences after massive overdosage returned to normal within 12 hours. Flashbacks (brief recurrences of some components of the LSD 'trip') may occur unpredictably up to a year later.

Reference

Kulig K. LSD. *Emerg Med Clin North Am* 1990; **8**: 551–558.

'Magic' mushrooms

General considerations

In recent years in the UK, there has been an annual spate of enquiries to poison information centres regarding the ingestion of 'magic' mushrooms. These are hallucinogenic species eaten for 'kicks' with *Psilocybe semilanceata*, the liberty cap mushroom, being most commonly involved. They are found in September and October in parks, football pitches and golf courses amongst other places and are eaten mainly by young teenagers. The optimal number necessary for a 'trip' is very much a matter of trial and error. Inevitably some individuals become poisoned.

Features

The features of poisoning can be classified into three groups – distorted perception, behavioural changes and physical effects. Perception is distorted in much the same way as with cannabis (p. 86) and individuals react to this in a variety of ways, some becoming aggressive and violent while others sit immobile looking vacant. The physical effects include vomiting, abdominal pain, dilated pupils and slight increases in blood pressure.

Management

Gastric emptying is probably unnecessary. Activated charcoal may be given but there is no objective evidence of its efficacy. Sedation should only rarely be necessary and most patients can be allowed to sleep off the effects. Ability to judge heights and distances may be impaired for some days and appropriate advice about driving and the use of machinery is indicated.

Mefenamic acid

General considerations

Overdosage (accidental and deliberate) with this widely prescribed analgesic is common in the UK. One case of intravenous administration has been reported.

Features

Convulsions are the most serious feature and occur in the 10–20% of patients who have the highest plasma mefenamic acid concentrations. They are often preceded by muscle twitching, are usually brief and do not recur. Occasionally, however, they may be more frequent. Vomiting and diarrhoea may develop.

Management

Repeated doses of activated charcoal should be given. Diazepam may be required for repeated convulsions but other symptomatic measures are rarely required. Complete recovery can be expected within 12 hours.

Plasma mefenamic acid concentrations

Plasma mefenamic acid concentrations of up to 462 mg/l have been reported after overdosage (therapeutic concentrations are approximately 10 mg/l). Like ibuprofen, the plasma half-life, even after overdosage, is very short (2–3 hours).

References

McKillop G, Canning GP. A case of intravenous and oral mefenamic acid poisoning. *Scot Med J* 1987; **32**: 81–82.

Smolinske SC, Hall AH, Vandenberg SA *et al.* Toxic effects of nonsteroidal anti-inflammatory drugs in overdose. *Drug Saf* 1990; **5**: 252–274.

Meprobamate

General considerations

Meprobamate enjoyed considerable popularity as a tranquillizer in the 1950s and 1960s, before it was ousted by the benzodiazepines. It shares many of the pharmacological properties of barbiturates. Regular use induces hepatic microsomal enzymes and tolerance and acute withdrawal of large doses (>2 g/day) results in an abstinence syndrome.

Features

The features of acute meprobamate poisoning are the same as those of barbiturate overdosage (p. 75). In uncomplicated cases coma seldom lasts longer than 36 hours though occasional deaths have been recorded.

Management

The majority of patients require no more than supportive care. Repeated oral charcoal should then be given.

Measures to increase elimination of meprobamate are only indicated when urgent recovery of consciousness is desirable or the patient is very severely poisoned. There is no merit in attempting forced diuresis. Haemodialysis removes significant amounts of meprobamate but charcoal haemoperfusion is even more efficient and is preferred. Patients should satisfy the criteria on p. 51 before these techniques are used.

Plasma meprobamate concentrations

Plasma meprobamate concentrations must be measured by a specific method such as gas chromatography. Non-tolerant patients would be expected to be unconscious with levels exceeding 50 mg/l though values of up to 300 mg/l may be encountered after acute poisoning. The plasma half-life is about 15 hours.

References

Eeckhout E, Huyghens L, Loef B *et al*. Meprobamate poisoning, hypotension and the Swan-Ganz catheter. *Intens Care Med* 1988; **14**: 437–438.
Jacobsen D, Wiik-Larsen E, Saltvedt E *et al*. Meprobamate kinetics during and after terminated hemoperfusion in acute intoxications. *Clin Toxicol* 1987; **25**: 317–331.

Mercury (inorganic)

General considerations

Acute inorganic mercury poisoning has occurred after ingestion of mercury salts, particularly mercuric chloride, accidental and deliberate injection of metallic mercury, inhalation of mercury vapour when thermometers or barometers have broken in heated ovens and inhalation of metallic mercury from ruptured bougie bags. Fortunately, the commonest accidental exposure to mercury, the ingestion of the bulbs of clinical thermometers by children, does not lead to poisoning since insignificant quantities are absorbed from the gastrointestinal tract.

Features

The features of inorganic mercury poisoning depend to some extent on the route of exposure.

Ingestion of a single large dose of mercurous chloride (calomel) does not usually cause symptoms since it is poorly absorbed. In contrast the gastrointestinal effects of mercuric chloride have earned this salt the name 'corrosive sublimate'. It produces a corrosive haemorrhagic gastroenteritis with severe vomiting and profuse watery diarrhoea (both of which may contain blood) associated with abdominal cramps, limb muscle pain and shock. Acute renal failure due to a direct effect of mercury on the renal tubule is invariable with severe poisoning.

Inhalation of air containing high mercury vapour concentrations produces symptoms within an hour including cough, chest pain, breathlessness due to an acute pneumonitis, shivering, generalized weakness, anorexia and joint pains. Less acute exposure by the same route leads to nausea, salivation, headache, irritability, fatigue, memory impairment, sleeplessness and incoordination in the upper limbs – the usual features of chronic mercurialism.

An acute inflammatory reaction occurs at the site of subcutaneous injection of metallic mercury but the degree of systemic toxicity is variable. Some patients have no features of poisoning while others become febrile, have muscular spasms, stomatitis, abdominal pain, and progress to renal failure and death. Embolization of mercury to the lungs may complicate subcutaneous as well as intravenous injection of metallic mercury. Symptoms following the latter also vary.

Inhaled globules of mercury are usually walled off by granulomatous tissue.

Management

Treatment for swallowed broken thermometer bulbs is unnecessary.

Gastric emptying is contraindicated after ingestion of mercuric chloride because of the corrosive actions on the stomach. Fluid balance must be carefully monitored and renal failure treated conventionally. Analgesics may be required for pain.

Individuals should be evacuated immediately if the atmosphere is contaminated by mercury vapour.

Surgical excision of subcutaneous metallic mercury should be undertaken to minimize both the local reaction and the risk of systemic poisoning. The completeness of drainage is readily assessed radiologically.

Chelation therapy should be given promptly when features of systemic poisoning develop, regardless of the route of exposure. The drug of choice is dimercaprol (British Anti-Lewisite, BAL) in a maximum dose of 4 mg/kg 4-hourly for 2 days followed by 3 mg/kg twice daily for 8 days. Penicillamine may also be of value though its role in acute mercury poisoning has not been assessed.

References

Aguado S, de Quiros IF, Marin R *et al*. Acute mercury vapour intoxication: report of six cases. *Nephrol Dial Transplant* 1989; **4**: 133–136.

Kostyniak PJ, Greizerstein HB, Goldstein J *et al*. Extracorporeal regional complexing haemodialysis treatment of acute inorganic mercury intoxication. *Hum Exp Toxicol* 1990; **9**: 137–141.

Murray KM, Hedgepeth JC. Intravenous self-administration of metallic mercury: efficacy of dimercaprol therapy. *Drug Intell Clin Pharmacol* 1988; **22**: 972–975.

Sauder P, Livardjani F, Jaeger A *et al*. Acute mercury chloride intoxication. Effects of hemodialysis and plasma exchange on mercury kinetic. *J Toxicol Clin Toxicol* 1988; **26**: 189–197.

Metaldehyde

General considerations

Metaldehyde (metacetaldehyde) is widely available to the public in the form of pellets used for killing slugs. Less frequently it is used as a solid fuel. It is poorly soluble in water.

Features

Small children and animals are most at risk from accidental poisoning but this is rarely serious. Any quantity is likely to give gastrointestinal symptoms while more than 100 mg/kg body weight may cause serious toxicity.

Nausea, vomiting, abdominal pain and diarrhoea often occur after a latent period of 1–3 hours. Severe poisoning is associated with a generalized increase in muscle tone, convulsions, impairment of consciousness and metabolic acidosis. Features of hepatic and renal tubular necrosis may become apparent after 2–3 days.

Management

The stomach should be emptied if more than 50 mg/kg has been ingested within 4 hours. Treatment thereafter is symptomatic including protection of the airway, control of convulsions and correction of the acid–base disturbance.

Reference

Longstreth WT, Pierson DJ. Metaldehyde poisoning from slug bait ingestion. *West J Med* 1982; **137**: 134–137.

Methanol

General considerations

Methanol (methyl or wood alcohol) is widely used in industry and laboratories as a solvent and is present in toxicologically insignificant concentrations (5%) in methylated and surgical spirits which are composed mainly of ethanol. It is also used as a windscreen-washer fluid. Although poisoning may occur from inhalation of methanol fumes or percutaneous absorption, ingestion is by far the commonest route. Many isolated cases of methanol self-poisoning occur in people who have access to the chemical at work but several epidemics have been reported when illicit alcohol has been adulterated with methanol, or methanol has been taken as an ethanol substitute.

Methanol is metabolized mainly in the liver by alcohol and acetaldehyde dehydrogenases to formaldehyde and formic acid. The rate of metabolism is independent of the plasma concentration and is only about one-seventh as rapid as that of ethanol. More than 50 ml methanol may cause features in adults but toxicity is due to its metabolites rather than the parent compound.

Diagnosis

The comments made in respect of the difficulty in making a diagnosis of ethylene glycol ingestion in the absence of an appropriate history (p. 121) apply equally to methanol. Urgent measurement of the plasma methanol concentration is indicated if the suspicion is raised but if this is not possible, with the exceptions of hypocalcaemia and crystalluria, the diagnostic clues discussed under ethylene glycol (p. 121) should be sought.

Features

Because of the slow rate of production of formaldehyde and formic acid there is frequently a latent period of about 12 hours between ingestion and the onset of symptoms, although occasionally the delay may be as long as 72 hours if ethanol is consumed concomitantly or after.

Conscious patients complain of headache, weakness, breathlessness and visual symptoms (usually dim or blurred vision and flashing lights). Violent attacks of abdominal colic are common and nausea and vomiting occur in about 50% of cases. Only a minority develop diarrhoea.

The patient often appears pale, apprehensive and restless. Sweating is common but the pulse rate and blood pressure are seldom abnormal till late in the course of the poisoning. Some pass through a phase of excitement before drowsiness and coma supervene. Convulsions occasionally occur.

Visual acuity may be reduced to perception of light or complete blindness. The pupils are usually dilated and unresponsive to light. Hyperaemia of the optic disc is the commonest abnormality on retinoscopy in the acute stage and subsides over 2–7 days. Peripapillary oedema often occurs but it develops more slowly and persists longer (up to 8 weeks). Venous engorgement and retinal haemorrhages are uncommon.

The abdomen is often rigid. Severe metabolic acidosis is common but Kussmaul's respiration is found in only 25% of cases. Bradycardia is a concomitant of respiratory failure and death follows progressive reduction of cardiac output, respiratory rate and tidal volume.

Cerebral oedema, necrosis in the putamen and haemorrhagic pancreatitis may be found at autopsy.

Plasma methanol concentrations

Plasma methanol concentrations are measured by gas–liquid chromatography. Levels in excess of 5 g/l have been reported.

Management

Supportive
The stomach should be emptied if more than 20 ml of methanol has been ingested by an adult, if any quantity has been taken by a child or if the patient is unconscious. Arterial blood gas analysis and aggressive correction of metabolic acidosis with intravenous sodium bicarbonate are essential if ocular toxicity is to be minimized. Convulsions should be controlled with diazepam.

Ethanol administration

As in ethylene glycol poisoning, ethanol should be given to compete with methanol as a substrate for alcohol dehydrogenase, thereby reducing the rate of formation of formaldehyde and formic acid. The mode of use is given on p. 122. Oral administration is only appropriate for minor intoxication. In severe poisoning ethanol should always be given intravenously and continued until the plasma methanol concentration is less than about 200 mg/l.

Haemodialysis

Haemodialysis removes methanol and its metabolites and, if started early enough, may prevent death and permanent visual damage. Dialysis is indicated for severe metabolic acidosis, if mental or visual symptoms attributable to the poison are present or plasma methanol concentrations exceed 500 mg/l, and should be continued till the concentration falls below 250 mg/l.

Prognosis

Severe methanol poisoning is frequently fatal and bradycardia, hypotension and severe acidosis are poor prognostic signs. The commonest long-term sequel is visual impairment, usually central scotomas or complete blindness secondary to optic atrophy. Patients who have gross visual symptoms or signs on presentation are unlikely to improve. Prevention of ocular damage depends on early correction of acidosis, administration of ethanol and removal of methanol and, more importantly, its toxic metabolites.

References

Jacobsen D, McMartin KE. Methanol and ethylene glycol poisonings. *Med Toxicol* 1986; **1**: 309–334.

Mahieu P, Hassoun A, Lauwerys R. Predictors of methanol intoxication with unfavourable outcome. *Hum Toxicol* 1989; **8**: 135–137.

Meatherall R, Krahn J. Excess serum osmolality gap after ingestion of methanol. *Clin Chem* 1990; **36**: 2004–2007.

Methylene chloride

General considerations

Methylene chloride (dichloromethane) is a widely used solvent commonly available in paints and paint strippers. Prolonged contact with tissues leads to local necrosis but systemic toxicity is usually due to inhalation subsequent upon use in enclosed and inadequately ventilated spaces. Some methylene chloride is metabolized by the cytochrome oxidase system to carbon monoxide but carboxyhaemoglobin concentrations do not commonly exceed 15% although exceptional cases with values of over 50% have been reported. Metabolism to carbon monoxide may continue for several hours after exposure has stopped but it is generally accepted that toxicity is more due to the direct effects of the parent compound than its metabolites.

Features

The major systemic effect is impairment of consciousness leading to coma. Multisystem abnormalities have also been reported including abdominal pain, joint pains, rashes and disturbed liver function tests. Prolonged skin exposure to high concentrations may produce severe burns and similar lesions occur in the oesophagus after ingestion. Rarely, inhalation of high concentrations may cause pulmonary oedema.

Management

Treatment is supportive. The patient should be removed from the toxic atmosphere or have contaminated clothing removed and the skin washed as appropriate. Gastric emptying is contraindicated after ingestion. Ensure a clear airway and adequate ventilation and correct acid–base abnormalities as required. High inspired oxygen concentrations are indicated particularly if carboxyhaemoglobin concentrations are raised.

Recently, hyperbaric oxygen has been used in a few cases but its value is uncertain and it did not prevent the postexposure increase in carboxyhaemoglobin levels in one patient. However, it may have a role in very severe poisoning with high levels.

Skin lesions should be treated as burns.

Reference

Leikin JB, Kaufman D, Lipscomb JW *et al*. Methylene chloride: report of five exposures and two deaths. *Am J Emerg Med* 1990; **8**: 534–537.

Metoclopramide

General considerations

Serious problems with metoclopramide overdosage have not been reported. However the drug not infrequently causes adverse reactions which patients find particularly frightening.

Features

The typical patient is a young woman who has been prescribed metoclopramide for hyperemesis gravidarum and presents with a dystonic reaction, usually in the form of uncontrollable chewing movements of the mouth and tongue, spasmodic torticollis or oculo-gyric crises. Consciousness is not impaired.

Management

Obviously no further metoclopramide should be given. The patient should be reassured. Intramuscular diphenhydramine (2 mg/kg body weight to a maximum of 50 mg), procyclidine (5–10 mg for an adult) or benztropine (1–2 mg for an adult) will abolish the dystonic reactions within a few minutes.

Mianserin

General considerations

Mianserin is a tetracyclic antidepressant which lacks the anticholinergic properties of tricyclic antidepressants and maprotiline. Acute mianserin overdosage is probably not as uncommon as the scant literature on the subject might lead one to believe and that may simply reflect the unremarkable consequences in most cases.

Features

Drowsiness has been the most common feature in poisoned adults but the few patients reported to have been unconscious had taken additional CNS depressants. Hypertension has been found as frequently as hypotension and though dysrhythmias have not been detected, one patient had first degree heart block which reverted to normal as the plasma mianserin concentration fell. In contrast to overdosage with tricyclic antidepressants and maprotiline, convulsions have not yet been reported with mianserin poisoning although the drug may have epileptogenic properties.

Management

Repeated doses of oral charcoal should be given. Treatment is symptomatic and supportive. Haemodialysis was used to treat one patient who had a plasma mianserin concentration of 780 µg/l 5 hours after ingestion but it failed to alter the rate of elimination of the drug and was obviously ineffective.

Mistletoe

General considerations

It is not uncommon for young children to eat mistletoe berries. There are two plants known by this common name; the European *Viscum album* and the North American *Phoradendron tomentosum* whose toxic principles are known as viscotoxin and phoratoxin respectively. They are long chain polypeptides which cause progressive depolarization of muscle cell membranes, perhaps by binding to membrane sites normally occupied by calcium. Fortunately, they do not appear to be present in the berries, the part of the plant most commonly ingested. The ingestion of up to three berries or leaves is thought unlikely to cause features whereas drinking teas made from *Phoradendron tomentosum* has produced serious poisoning.

Features

Though the potential for serious poisoning is considerable, children seldom eat sufficient berries to develop symptoms. Vomiting, abdominal pain and diarrhoea are the commonest features amongst those who do. Very rarely there may be muscle weakness, bradycardia and circulatory failure.

Management

Children who have eaten only 1–3 berries or leaves do not require hospital admission. Those who have taken more should be observed and given activated charcoal. Other measures depend on clinical developments. Calcium gluconate may be worth trying if circulatory failure develops since calcium has been shown experimentally to reverse the effects of viscotoxins on muscle cells.

Reference

Hall AH, Spoerke DG, Rumack BH. Assessing mistletoe toxicity. *Ann Emerg Med* 1986; **15**: 1320–1323.

Monoamine oxidase inhibitors

Phenelzine   Tranylcypromine

General considerations

Acute overdosage with monoamine oxidase inhibitors is uncommon but the consequences are frequently serious or even fatal. The features of poisoning are due to secondary tissue accumulation of catecholamines rather than to a direct toxic effect of the drug.

Features

There is commonly a latent period of 6–12 hours before tissue catecholamine concentrations increase sufficiently to cause toxicity.

Most features are the result of CNS overactivity. Initially there is a feeling of unease followed by increasing agitation, hallucinations and restlessness. Motor activity may increase to such an extent that the patient performs 'continuous gymnastics' with writhing of the limbs and trunk, grimacing and grinding of the teeth. Muscle tone is often greatly increased, occasionally to such a degree that opisthotonus develops. The limb reflexes are exaggerated with extensor plantar responses. Myoclonus and convulsions are common. Marked pyrexia, disproportionate to the degree of muscular activity, may be present. Not surprisingly, rhabdomyolysis and acute renal failure are potential complications. The pupils are usually dilated and may be unresponsive to light. Other ocular features include nystagmus and 'ping-pong' gaze (rhythmic pendular conjugate deviation of the eyes in the horizontal plane from one extreme to the other). Tachycardia, increased blood pressure and profuse sweating are common.

Management

It is advisable to observe any patient who has taken an overdose of monoamine oxidase inhibitors for a minimum of 12 hours for the onset of toxic features.

Treatment is mainly supportive. Repeated doses of oral activated charcoal should be given if possible. Haloperidol or chlorpromazine may help reduce overactivity and though there are no reports of the use of beta-adrenoceptor blockers in this type of poisoning they should be effective if given in large enough doses. Tepid sponging or ice-packs may be required to prevent hyperpyrexia reaching dangerous heights. Dantrolene is indicated if the increase in muscle tone is extreme. If convulsions are frequent, curarization and assisted ventilation may be more appropriate than administration of anticonvulsants.

It has been claimed that haemodialysis is effective but laboratory evidence to support this has not been presented. Alpha-adrenoceptor blockade with phentolamine and phenoxybenzamine proved useful in one case but is only recommended with invasive haemodynamic monitoring.

References

Breheny FX, Dobb GJ, Clarke GM. Phenelzine poisoning. *Anaesthesia* 1986; **41**: 53–56.

Mallampalli R, Pentel PR, Anderson DC. Nonreactive pupils due to monoamine oxidase inhibitor overdose. *Crit Care Med* 1987; **15**: 536–537.

Verrilli MR, Salanga VD, Kozachuk WE *et al.* Phenelzine toxicity responsive to dantrolene. *Neurology* 1987; **37**: 865–867.

Watkins HC, Ellis CJK. Ping pong gaze in reversible coma due to overdose of monoamine oxidase inhibitor. *J Neurol Neurosurg Psychiatry* 1989; **52**: 539.

Mushrooms

General considerations

Of the numerous known genera of fungi it is estimated that some 50 are harmful to humans, although about 90% of fatalities are due to one variety, *Amanita phalloides* (the death cap mushroom). The distribution of individual species of fungi varies considerably from one country to another and even within any given country depending on its growth requirements. The constituent toxins may also vary to some extent.

Present-day concern about mushroom poisoning arises from the increasing trend to pick and eat wild varieties as part of the vogue for a return to a more 'natural' diet or a search for a hallucinogenic 'trip' (see p. 145). However, the differentiation of poisonous from edible types is not nearly as easy as some suggest and inevitably toxic species are ingested. Since doctors are seldom any wiser in matters of identification than most of their patients, it is fortunate that the number of fungi which cause serious illness is so small and that the nature of their toxins and the type and time course of the symptoms they produce are reasonably well-defined. In most cases, however, the mechanisms of toxicity are not known.

When taking the history from someone poisoned with mushrooms attention should be paid to:

1 The interval between ingestion and onset of symptoms, which is crucial in distinguishing between non-serious and potentially fatal poisoning.
2 The number of different varieties of mushrooms eaten. This is important because edible and poisonous types often grow in close proximity.
3 Whether or not alcohol was drunk between eating the mushrooms and the onset of symptoms.

4 Whether or not the fungi were cooked before eating. Some toxins (e.g. haemolysins and some gastrointestinal irritants) are inactivated by heat while others (particularly those with more serious effects) are thermostable.

If possible, specimens of the mushrooms should be identified by an expert mycologist.

Features

It is diagnostically and prognostically most valuable to consider the initial features in relation to the time interval since ingestion, as shown in Table 4.3. In general, the sooner symptoms start, the less serious the poisoning, although this may not be the case if a mixture of species has been ingested.

Gastrointestinal irritation of early onset usually lasts only a few hours and is seldom severe enough to cause serious dehydration except occasionally in small children. Similarly visual hallucinations do not usually persist longer than 4–6 hours but there are reports of some patients having distortion of perception lasting several days or psychiatric symptoms for weeks.

In mild cases of *Gyromitra* poisoning symptoms usually settle over 6 days but acute hepatocellular necrosis with its potentially lethal complications may develop in severe cases.

By far the most serious mushroom poisoning is that caused by *Amanita phalloides* and the related species *A. verna* and *A. virosa*. After a latent period of about 12 hours there is usually nausea, severe vomiting and profuse watery diarrhoea comparable to that seen in cholera. These features may subside gradually over several hours and a phase of apparent recovery lasting up to 48–72 hours after ingestion ensues. Evidence of massive hepatic necrosis may then appear and acute renal failure may also develop. The mortality in this phase is high. About 20% of survivors may progress to chronic liver disease.

Coprine, the toxic principle of the common ink cap, is converted in the body to L-aminocyclopropanol which inhibits alcohol dehydrogenase. Ingestion of alcohol then causes accumulation of acetaldehyde and symptoms identical to the alcohol–disulfiram reaction.

Management

The stomach should be emptied if the patient presents within 4 hours unless identification of the mushrooms or the nature of the symptoms indicates that poisoning is mild and is unlikely to become worse.

Table 4.3 Ingestion/presentation interval and features of poisoning with mushrooms

Interval	Initial features	Toxins	Fungi	Treatment for severe symptoms
	Nausea, vomiting, diarrhoea	Undetermined gastrointestinal irritants	Numerous fungi including *Entoloma sinuatum*, *Boletus satanas*, *Nalonea sericea*, *Paxillus involutus*, *Agaricus xanthedermus*, *Russula* species, *Tricholoma* species among others	Antiemetics, intravenous fluids, correction of electrolyte imbalance
2 hours or less	Profuse sweating, salivation, vomiting, abdominal colic, diarrhoea, rhinorrhoea, blurred vision	Muscarine	Species of *Clitocybe* and *Inocybe*	Atropine
	Hallucinations without impairment of consciousness	Psilocybin Psilocin	Species of *Psilocybe* and *Panaeolus* including the liberty cap (*Psilocybe semilanceata*)	Reassurance and sedation with diazepam or chlorpromazine
	Hallucinations with impaired consciousness	Ibotenic acid Muscimol	*Amanita muscaria* (fly agaric) and *A. pantherina* (panther cap)	
6 hours or more	Very sudden-onset headache, dizziness, tiredness, abdominal pain, vomiting	Gyromitrin (hydrolyses to monomethylhydrazine)	*Gyromitra esculenta* (brain fungus)	See text
12 hours (approx)	Severe vomiting, abdominal cramp, profuse watery diarrhoea	Amanatins (cyclic octapeptides)	*Amanita phalloides* (death cap), *A. verna*, *A. virosa* and some species of *Galerina*	See text
Up to 24 hours	Flushing, sweating, nausea immediately after alcohol consumption	Coprine (active form 1-amino-cyclopropanol)	*Coprinus atramentarius* (common ink cap)	Propranolol
72 hours or more	Thirst, polyuria leading to renal failure	Unspecified polypeptides	*Cortinarius* species	Conventional measures for renal failure

The majority of patients with early symptoms will not require specific measures but, if severe, appropriate treatment should be given as indicated in Table 4.3.

When hepatotoxic and nephrotoxic species have been ingested, careful monitoring of liver and renal function is mandatory as in paracetamol poisoning (p. 173) and prophylactic measures against hepatic encephalopathy should be instituted on the earliest evidence of hepatic damage. In the early stages adequate replacement of fluid and electrolytes lost by vomiting and diarrhoea is essential and antiemetics such as metoclopramide (10 mg intramuscularly for an adult) may be helpful.

The more specific treatment of *A. phalloides*-type poisoning is a matter of considerable debate. Most of the support for particular forms of treatment is anecdotal rather than objective and is, no doubt, in large part due to the difficulty of predicting the outcome without treatment in individual cases. Regular oral activated charcoal has been recommended to interrupt enterohepatic circulation of the toxins and at least has the merit of being harmless. Penicillin and silibinin are considered to protect against the actions of amanitins, one of the two groups of toxins present in *Amanita* species. Penicillin G should therefore be given in a dose of 300 000–1 000 000 units/kg body weight per day and silibinin (if available) in a dose of 20–50 mg/kg per day. Thioctic acid may increase rather than decrease mortality.

Not surprisingly, haemodialysis and charcoal haemoperfusion have been tried but there is no objective evidence that they remove significant quantities of toxin or improve the prognosis. Animal studies indicate that amanitins cannot be detected in the plasma 5 hours after an intravenous dose, having been taken up by tissues or excreted in the urine during that time. Clearly measures aimed at increasing elimination would have to be implemented at a very early stage if there was to be any hope of removing significant quantities.

Patients who develop hepatic encephalopathy should be considered for liver transplantation.

References

Benjamin DR. Mushroom poisoning in infants and children: the *Amanita pantherina/ muscaria* group. *Clin Toxicol* 1992; **30**: 13–22.

Bouget J, Bousser J, Pats B *et al*. Acute renal failure following collective intoxication by *Cortinarius orellanus*. *Intens Care Med* 1990; **16**: 506–510.

Olesen LL. Amatoxin intoxication. *Scand J Urol Nephrol* 1990; **24**: 231–234.

Pinson CW, Daya MR, Benner KG *et al*. Liver transplantation for severe *Amanita phalloides* mushroom poisoning. *Am J Surg* 1990; **159**: 493–499.

Stollard D, Edes TE. Muscarinic poisoning from medications and mushrooms. *Postgrad Med J* 1989; **85**: 341–345.

Nicotine

General considerations

Nicotine ingestion, in the form of tobacco and nicotine-containing chewing gum, is not uncommon amongst children. Most who consume 1 cigarette or 3 cigarette ends will have toxic features.

Features

Vomiting and nausea are amongst the most common features and may be associated with agitation, hyperactivity and tachycardia. Abdominal pain, drowsiness, muscle weakness and jerking of the limbs are less common. Rarely, there may be convulsions, respiratory depression and dysrhythmias. Chronic nicotine gum use by adults has been reported to cause atrial fibrillation.

Management

Children who have ingested potentially toxic amounts (as defined above) should be referred to hospital. Gastric emptying by lavage has been recommended if more than 5 whole cigarettes, 8 stubs or 5 pieces of gum have been ingested but there is no evidence that it is of value. Induced emesis is best avoided because of the risk of convulsions. Activated charcoal should be given. Further treatment should be unnecessary but symptomatic measures may be required.

References

Borys DJ, Setzer SC, Ling LJ. CNS depression in an infant after the ingestion of tobacco. *Vet Hum Toxicol* 1988; **30**: 20–22.
Lavoie FW, Harris TM. Fatal nicotine ingestion. *J Emerg Med* 1991; **9**: 133–136.
Smolinske SC, Spoerke DG, Spiller SK *et al.* Cigarette and nicotine chewing gum toxicity in children. *Hum Toxicol* 1988; **7**: 27–31.

Non-steroidal anti-inflammatory drugs

General considerations

Mefenamic acid and ibuprofen are by far the most common of the non-steroidal anti-inflammatory drugs taken in acute overdosage and are considered separately on pages 146 and 131 respectively. Information on overdosage with other members of this large group of drugs is scarce.

Features

Fenoprofen and naproxen in overdosage appear to cause similar effects to mefenamic acid with seizures and metabolic acidosis as the principal features. Maternal poisoning with naproxen 8 hours before delivery caused hyponatraemia and fluid retention in the neonate.

Management

Management is as for mefenamic acid (p. 146).

References

Alun-Jones E, Williams J. Hyponatremia and fluid retention in a neonate associated with maternal naproxen overdosage. *Clin Toxicol* 1986; **24**: 257–260.

Kolodzik JM, Eilers MA, Angelos MG. Nonsteroidal anti-inflammatory drugs and coma: a case report of fenoprofen overdose. *Ann Emerg Med* 1990; **19**: 378–381.

Martinez R, Smith DW, Frankel LR. Severe metabolic acidosis after acute naproxen sodium ingestion. *Ann Emerg Med* 1989; **18**: 1102–1104.

Opioid analgesics

Buprenorphine	Etorphine	Opium
Codeine	Heroin (diamorphine)	Oxymorphone
Dextromoramide	Hydromorphone	Papaveretum
Dextropropoxyphene	Meptazinol	Pentazocine
Dihydrocodeine	Methadone	Phenazocine
Diphenoxylate	Morphine	Pethidine (meperidine)
Dipipanone	Nalbuphine	

General considerations

Opium is derived from the milky fluid which exudes from the cut surface of unripe seed-capsules of *Papaver somniferum*. It contains a number of alkaloids of which the phenanthrene compounds, morphine and codeine, are the most important. Over the years a number of related narcotic drugs have been derived from these, or synthesized (opioids). They are extensively used as potent analgesics, euphoriants, antitussives and antidiarrhoeal agents.

Codeine is a constituent of many over-the-counter analgesics commonly taken in overdosage but its effects are usually (but not always) overshadowed by those of salicylates or paracetamol, the major constituents of such preparations. Self-poisoning with combined preparations of dextropropoxyphene (propoxyphene) and paracetamol are now much less common than previously, although still posing potentially serious problems.

Poisoning with morphine, heroin and methadone is usually the result of accidental intravenous overdosage by drug addicts due to the unpredictable potency of 'street' drugs. There are therefore likely to be marked differences in the incidence of this type of opioid poisoning, being a much larger problem in selected quarters of large cities than in rural areas. Street drugs are commonly adulterated with any of a number of substances which are usually inert and do not contribute to mortality. Dextromoramide and dipipanone are encountered only rarely now but dihydrocodeine and buprenorphine are popular with addicts, particularly the latter because of its ready solubility in water. It seems likely that many doctors who prescribe these drugs do not appreciate that they are opioid analgesics with the same potential for misuse as morphine and heroin. Prolonged use induces tolerance and profound psychological and physical dependence.

Poisoning with other opioids is infrequent but two merit special mention. Diphenoxylate overdosage is not uncommon among children who eat Lomotil tablets (diphenoxylate and atropine) prescribed for treatment of diarrhoea. Etorphine is about 400 times more potent than morphine in humans and is used in veterinary medicine for immobilizing large animals. Severe poisoning from both accidental and deliberate self-injection has been reported.

Features

Coma, pinpoint pupils and marked reduction of the respiratory rate are the hallmarks of poisoning with opioid analgesics. The depth of respiration may also be reduced but in some cases it may seem normal or even increased. Respiratory arrest, hypotension and hypothermia are common in severe poisoning. Convulsions may occur, particularly in children. The presence of injection marks or venous tracking in an unconscious patient indicates that he or she is an addict and should arouse suspicion of opioid overdosage. Pulmonary oedema is a potentially lethal complication of mainlining opioid analgesics and though relatively uncommon in clinical practice, it is frequently found in those who die. Cardiac contractility may be impaired by propoxyphene metabolites or hypoxic damage.

The speed with which features of poisoning develop clearly depends on the dose and the route by which it is taken, being faster after intravenous than after oral administration. However, concern has been expressed at the alarming rapidity with which dextropropoxyphene taken orally can produce severe coma, convulsions and fatal respiratory depression. Deaths have occurred within an hour of taking the overdose.

It is not sufficiently appreciated that individuals taking preparations containing dextropropoxyphene may not survive long enough to reach medical care. This should be borne in mind when prescribing some popular analgesics to patients at risk of self-poisoning.

Management

Supportive

Even if an opioid antagonist is immediately available steps should be taken to ensure a clear airway and to support respiration if necessary. However, the need for endotracheal intubation and assisted ventilation can be obviated by the prompt administration of adequate doses of naloxone. When CNS depression has been reversed, the stomach should be emptied. The time limit for this procedure should be extended to 6 hours since opiates greatly delay gastric emptying.

Naloxone – use in non-addicts

Actions. Naloxone is a specific opioid antagonist which has none of the partial agonist effects of nalorphine. It is the only antagonist which reverses the effects of pentazocine overdosage but even very large doses are unlikely to counteract those of buprenorphine. With other opioids, however, administration causes the pupils to dilate, the respiratory rate and minute volume to rise (often transiently overshooting normal), consciousness returns and hypotension is reversed. The response is dramatic and it is not uncommon for intubated patients to sit up and extubate themselves.

Initial dosage. The optimum initial dose depends on the severity of poisoning and the drug taken and for an adult is usually at least 1.2 mg intravenously (0.4 mg for a child). Smaller doses of naloxone (e.g. 0.4 mg intravenously for an adult) are adequate for reversing the effects of therapeutic doses but are useless in the presence of a large opioid overdose because they are insufficient to compete effectively at receptor sites.

Routes of administration. While intravenous administration is optimum, there are occasions when venous access is not possible. In such situations naloxone may be instilled down an endotracheal tube or given intramuscularly. Injection sublingually has been used in shocked patients.

Duration of action and repeated doses. The effect of a single bolus of naloxone is short-lived and patients must be carefully observed for recurrence of coma and respiratory depression. Repeated doses of naloxone are almost always required and in some cases an intravenous infusion may be more appropriate. However, it cannot be emphasized too strongly that there is no fixed dosage schedule. The dose of naloxone must be titrated against the clinical response in each case and clinicians should not become faint-hearted if they have to exceed 'usual' doses. As much as 75 mg naloxone has been given in 24 hours without obvious adverse effects.

Adverse effects. Naloxone has been reported to cause pulmonary oedema and ventricular dysrhythmias but these do not occur sufficiently frequently to outweigh the enormous benefits of naloxone.

Naloxone – use in opioid addicts

Administration of naloxone to poisoned opioid addicts may precipitate an acute withdrawal syndrome comprising abdominal cramps, nausea, diarrhoea, piloerection and vasoconstriction. While this is distressing, it is short-lived and seldom as severe as the mass media (and the patients) would have one believe and is obviously not a contraindication to the use of naloxone for the treatment of serious opioid poisoning in addicts. More importantly, those whose intoxication is fully reversed by naloxone may immediately attempt to leave medical care while, because of the short half-life of the antidote, they are at risk of lapsing back into CNS depression. Their behaviour may also be troublesome at this time, particularly if they feel symptoms of withdrawal. Their management may therefore be made easier by titrating the amount of naloxone given so that life-threatening toxicity is reversed without rendering the patient fully conscious and mobile. Those who are capable of, and insist on, leaving should first be given an intramuscular dose of naloxone.

Naloxone – failure to respond to adequate doses

Failure to obtain a response to an adequate dose of naloxone is an indication to review the diagnosis. However an absent or partial response may still be consistent with a diagnosis of opioid overdosage if the patient has taken other CNS depressants or has suffered hypoxic brain damage before treatment.

Diagnostic use of naloxone

Naloxone is commonly regarded as being so safe that it is given extensively (by doctors and paramedics) in the absence of a certain diagnosis of opioid poisoning but the beneficial response rate is less than 10%, even in communities where abuse of opioids is high. While the indiscriminate use of naloxone as a therapeutic test for narcotic poisoning is not a substitute for intelligent appraisal of each poisoned patient, it would appear that there is more to gain than lose from arbitrary use of naloxone.

Unexpected responses to naloxone

While it is possible that naloxone occasionally reverses or partially reverses the CNS toxicity of ethanol, benzodiazepines, and, occasionally other drugs, in the UK and in patients who are not obviously addicts, an unexpected response raises the possibility of poisoning with a paracetamol/opioid formulation. The plasma paracetamol concentration should be measured urgently. Patients who have become unconscious from such combined preparations have also taken sufficient paracetamol to be at risk of severe, but preventable, liver necrosis (p. 172).

References

Bloor RN, Smalldridge NJF. Intravenous use of slow release morphine sulphate tablets. *Br Med J* 1990; **300**: 640–641.

Challoner KR, McCarron MM, Newton EJ. Pentazocine (Talwin) intoxication: report of 57 cases. *J Emerg Med* 1990; **8**: 67–74.

Davidson AG, Collinson PO, Assefi AR *et al*. Meptazinol overdose producing near fatal respiratory depression. *Hum Toxicol* 1987; **6**: 331.

Goldfrank L, Weisman RS, Errick JK. A dosing nomogram for continuous infusion of intravenous naloxone. *Ann Emerg Med* 1986; **15**: 566–570.

Leslie PJ, Dyson EH, Proudfoot AT. Opiate toxicity after self poisoning with aspirin and codeine. *Br Med J* 1986; **292**: 96.

McCarron MM, Challoner KR, Thompson GA. Diphenoxylate-atropine (Lomotil) overdose in children: an update (report of eight cases and review of the literature). *Pediatrics* 1991; **87**: 694–700.

Schwartz JA, Koenigsberg MD. Naloxone-induced pulmonary edema. *Ann Emerg Med* 1987; **16**: 1294–1296.

Shesser R, Jotte R, Olshaker J. The contribution of impurities to the acute morbidity of illegal drug use. *Am J Emerg Med* 1991; **9**: 336–342.

Smith F, Lee R, Haindl W. Hypoxic cardiomyopathy: acute myocardial dysfunction after severe hypoxia. *Aust NZ Med J* 1989; **19**: 488–492.

Strom J. Acute propoxyphene self-poisoning. *Dan Med Bull* 1989; **36**: 316–336.

Swadi H, Wells B, Power R. Misuse of dihydrocodeine tartrate (DF 118) among opiate addicts. *Br Med J* 1990; **300**: 1313.

Yealy DM, Paris PM, Kaplan RM *et al*. The safety of prehospital naloxone administration by paramedics. *Ann Emerg Med* 1990; **19**: 902–905.

Organophosphate and carbamate insecticides

Organophosphates

Azinphos methyl	Fonofos	Phoxim
Carbophenothion	Formothion	Pirimiphos ethyl
Chlorfenvinphos	Heptenophos	Pirimiphos methyl
Chlorpyrifos	Iodofenphos	Propetamphos
Demeton-s-methyl	Malathion	Pyrazophos
Diazinon	Mephosfolan	Quinalphos
Dichlorvos	Mevinphos	Thiometon
Dimethoate	Omethoate	Thionazin
Disulfoton	Oxydemeton-methyl	Triazophos
Ethoprophos	Phorate	Trichlorphon
Fenitrothion	Phosalone	Vamidothion

Carbamates

Aldicarb	Carbosulfan	Pirimicarb
Bendiocarb	Ethiofencarb	Propoxur
Benfuracarb	Methiocarb	Thiofanox
Carbaryl	Methomyl	
Carbofuran	Oxamyl	

General considerations

Organophosphate and carbamate insecticides are used extensively in agriculture and horticulture throughout the world. They are thought to be involved in about 3 million cases of human poisoning annually, particularly in developing countries, and to be the cause of about 40 000 deaths. Acute poisoning with these compounds occurs in a variety of ways. They are most commonly taken deliberately, usually by ingestion, although there are occasional reports of self-injection. Accidental poisoning is also common and outbreaks of poisoning have occurred when flour, vegetables and other foodstuffs have been contaminated. Children may swallow liquid formulations kept in the home but symptoms as a result of the domestic use of sprays are uncommon. Poisoning may also occur when these substances are being used for their proper purpose though the risk is negligible if the manufacturer's recommendations on preparation of solutions and safety precautions are heeded. Unfortunately, environmental factors, particularly high temperatures and humidity, encourage users to ignore wearing masks and protective clothing and risk poisoning by inhalation of spray or by percutaneous absorption. The latter usually results from failure to change soiled clothing immediately and from leaking spray equipment carried on the back as well as direct dermal contamination.

Organophosphates and carbamates act by inhibiting cholinesterases causing accumulation of acetylcholine at central and peripheral cholinergic nerve endings, including neuromuscular junctions. Some are directly toxic while others (e.g. malathion) have to be metabolized before being effective. Carbamates produce relatively short-lived inhibition of cholinesterase since the carbamate–enzyme complex tends to dissociate spontaneously. In contrast, the duration of inhibition by organophosphates varies considerably from one member of the class to another but, in general, is much longer than with carbamates. Three independent reactions determine the speed of onset and severity of poisoning:

1 The rate of phosphorylation of the enzyme which, in turn, depends on the affinity of the enzyme for the organophosphate, the concentration of the latter and the time available for the reaction.

2 The rate of spontaneous hydrolysis of the phosphorylated enzyme and release of active enzyme. (This is the process referred to by the term 'reactivation'.)
3 The rate of 'ageing' of the phosphorylated enzyme complex by a process of dealkylation of the organophosphate component. Once this happens, reactivation is impossible and recovery of cholinesterase activity depends on synthesis of new enzyme by the liver which may take days or weeks.

Features

Local
A garlic-like odour may be present from the poison. Skin exposed to organophosphate solutions for a few hours may become red and blistered. Accidental splashes in the eye will produce miosis and blurring of vision on the affected side.

Subclinical poisoning
Minor exposure may produce subclinical poisoning in which there is reduction of cholinesterase activity but no symptoms or signs.

Systemic poisoning
The speed of onset of symptoms depends on the route and magnitude of exposure. Inhalation and ingestion may produce local bronchial and gastrointestinal effects respectively within minutes but systemic features take longer to develop. However they are usually apparent within a few hours if a large dose is involved. The onset of systemic toxicity is slowest by the percutaneous route.

The features of organophosphate and carbamate poisoning are a blend of peripheral muscarinic effects of excess acetylcholine on the gastrointestinal tract, bronchi, heart, bladder and sweat, salivary and lachrymal glands; nicotinic actions at neuromuscular junctions and sympathetic ganglia; and CNS effects.

Mild poisoning is characterized by CNS stimulant effects including anxiety, restlessness, insomnia, nightmares, tiredness, dizziness, headache and muscarinic features such as nausea, vomiting, abdominal colic, diarrhoea, tenesmus, sweating, hypersalivation and chest tightness. Miosis may be present.

In addition to these symptoms, the patient who is moderately poisoned shows nicotinic effects, particularly muscle fasciculation, and generalized weakness sufficient to make walking impossible and speech difficult.

Consciousness is impaired in severe poisoning and there is widespread flaccid paresis of limb muscles (affecting proximal groups more than distal ones), respiratory muscles and (less commonly) various combinations of extraocular muscles. Patients who show severe muscle weakness early in the course of poisoning may have extensor plantar responses whereas those in whom paralytic features are delayed till about 24 hours after ingestion do not. The significance of this finding is not understood. Pulmonary oedema and cyanosis are common in severe poisoning and frothy secretions may pour from the mouth and nose, embarrassing respiration further. Convulsions may occur. Complete heart block, atrial fibrillation and other unspecified dysrhythmias have been reported infrequently.

Diagnosis

Clinical
In the absence of a history of exposure the diagnosis of organophosphate and carbamate poisoning may be very difficult. The prominent gastrointestinal symptoms with fever and polymorph leucocytosis may lead to an erroneous diagnosis of gastroenteritis. Miosis is an important diagnostic sign but in 10% or more of cases the diameter of the pupil is normal or even increased when nicotinic effects predominate. Similarly tachycardia and raised blood pressure are commoner than bradycardia and hypotension which occur late, if at all. Diagnosis may be further confused by the frequent finding of hyperglycaemia and glycosuria, though ketonuria is absent.

Plasma cholinesterase activity
Reduction of plasma cholinesterase activity confirms exposure to organophosphates or carbamate insecticides but values correlate poorly with the severity of poisoning. In subclinical poisoning activity may be reduced by up to 50%. Mild, moderate and severe acute poisoning are associated with reduction of cholinesterase activity to approximately 20–50%, 10–20% and <10% of normal respectively.

Management

The management of organophosphate poisoning involves supportive measures and administration of atropine to antagonize the muscarinic effects of excess acetylcholine and oximes to reactivate phosphorylated cholinesterase.

General
The removal of soiled clothing and thorough washing of contaminated skin with soap and water prevent further absorption. The stomach

should be emptied if the poison has been ingested. Activated charcoal may be given although there is no evidence that it is of value.

Blood should be taken for estimation of cholinesterase activity in every case, preferably before starting treatment. Red blood cell cholinesterase is usually the more sensitive but with some organophosphates (malathion and demeton-s-methyl) plasma cholinesterase is inhibited to a greater extent.

Treatment is unnecessary for subclinical poisoning but the patient should be kept under observation for about 24 hours to ensure that delayed toxicity does not develop.

Supportive measures

It must be emphasized that the patient who is severely poisoned by organophosphates or carbamates requires energetic supportive measures. Respiratory secretions must be effectively removed and endotracheal intubation may be necessary. Hypoxia must be corrected, particularly when large doses of atropine are being given. The adequacy of ventilation should be assessed by arterial blood gas analysis and assisted respiration started if necessary. Fluids lost by vomiting, diarrhoea and in pulmonary oedema should be replaced.

Atropine

Atropine is often the first drug and, regretfully, sometimes the only drug used in the treatment of symptomatic poisoning. Its major use is in reducing bronchorrhoea and bronchospasm. Adults should be given 2 mg intravenously every 10–30 min depending on the severity of poisoning till relief is obtained or signs of atropinization (flushed dry skin, tachycardia, dilated pupils and dry mouth) are obvious. The total dose required in the first 24 hours is commonly as much as 30 mg and occasionally much more is necessary. Children should be given 0.02 mg/kg body weight but may require up to 0.05 mg/kg. Not surprisingly, administration of such large doses in the absence of appropriate indications leads to atropine toxicity.

Oximes in carbamate intoxication

The use of oximes is contraindicated in carbamate poisoning.

Oximes in organophosphate intoxication

Oximes such as pralidoxime mesylate (P2S, 2-PAMM), pralidoxime chloride (2-PAM chloride, 2-PAMCl) or obidoxime (Toxogonin) reactivate phosphorylated cholinesterases provided they are given before the complex 'ages'. Pralidoxime is less toxic than obidoxime and should be given together with atropine to every symptomatic patient. The dose is 30 mg/kg body weight by slow intravenous injection. Its effects will usually be apparent within 30 min and include disappearance of convulsions and fasciculation, improvement in muscle power and recovery of consciousness. Further doses of the mesylate may be given 4-hourly and the chloride 6-hourly and may have to be given for several days in severe cases. Continuing clinical toxicity and measurement of cholinesterase activity may be used to guide the duration of therapy. Either salt of pralidoxime may be given in the same dose by the intramuscular route but this is inadvisable if treatment is likely to be prolonged. The administration of pralidoxime usually necessitates reduction of the amount of atropine given and may unmask atropine toxicity.

Diazepam
Diazepam (5–10 mg intravenously for an adult) will reduce anxiety and restlessness but larger doses (10–20 mg intravenously) may be required to control convulsions. Early use may reduce morbidity and mortality.

Prognosis

Mortality
Severe poisoning with organophosphates is usually fatal within 24 hours if untreated. Even with treatment a small proportion of cases die within days because of failure to respond significantly to adequate doses of atropine and pralidoxime. Mortality rates of up to 25% have been reported. Complete recovery should follow treatment of moderate and mild poisoning.

Intermediate syndrome
This is the term given to the development of cranial nerve and brainstem lesions together with a proximal neuropathy 1–4 days after acute intoxication. Respiratory failure secondary to muscle weakness is the most serious complication. The syndrome may persist for 2–3 weeks.

Late neuropathy
A longer-term consequence of acute poisoning is peripheral neuropathy due to axonal degeneration of large myelinated motor and sensory fibres. The lower limbs are particularly affected. This neuropathy characteristically starts 2–3 weeks after exposure and is thought to be caused by inhibition of neuropathy target esterase.

Ill-defined symptoms
These include tiredness, insomnia, inability to concentrate, depression and irritability.

References

Ballantyne B, Marrs TC. *Organophosphates and Carbamates*. Oxford: Butterworth-Heinemann, 1992.

de Kort WLAM, Kiestra SH, Sangster B. The use of atropine and oximes in organophosphate intoxications: a modified approach. *Clin Toxicol* 1988; **26**: 199–208.

de Wilde V, Vogelaers D, Colardyn F. Prompt recovery from severe cholinesterase-inhibitor poisoning - remarks on classification and therapy of organophosphate poisoning. *Klin Wochenschr* 1990; **68**: 615–618.

Goh KT, Yew FS, Ong KH *et al*. Acute organophosphorus food poisoning caused by contaminated green leafy vegetables. *Arch Environ Hlth* 1990; **45**: 180–184.

Kurtz PH. Pralidoxime in the treatment of carbamate intoxication. *Am J Emerg Med* 1990; **8**: 68–70.

Marques EGP. Acute intoxication by azinphos-ethyl. *J Anal Toxicol* 1990; **14**: 243–246.

Minton NA, Murray VSG. A review of organophosphate poisoning. *Med Toxicol* 1988; **3**: 350–375.

Sofer S, Tal A, Shahak E. Carbamate and organophosphate poisoning in early childhood. *Pediatr Emerg Care* 1989; **5**: 222–225.

Zwiener RJ, Ginsburg CM. Organophosphate and carbamate poisoning in infants and children. *Pediatrics* 1988; **81**: 121–126.

Paracetamol (acetaminophen)

General considerations

Paracetamol (acetaminophen) overdosage is currently the single most important cause of poisons information enquiries in the UK and is an increasing problem in the USA and other countries. It is now considerably more common than salicylate poisoning.

The toxicity of paracetamol in overdosage was first appreciated in 1966 when it was reported to cause jaundice and fatal hepatic necrosis. It soon became apparent that the liver damage was a dose-related effect. In therapeutic doses paracetamol is metabolized in the liver, largely to inactive sulphate and glucuronide conjugates. However, about 8% is converted into a highly toxic intermediate metabolite, N-acetyl-p-benzoquinone imine (NAPQI), which is normally immediately inactivated by conjugation with hepatic reduced glutathione and eventually excreted in the urine as cysteine and mercapturic acid conjugates. After overdosage increased amounts of NAPQI are formed and rapidly deplete the limited hepatic stores of glutathione. It is then free to bind irreversibly with macromolecules in the hepatocytes producing necrosis. There is clinical and experimental evidence that drugs which induce hepatic microsomal oxidases increase susceptibility to paracetamol toxicity by increasing the rate of production of the toxic metabolite. Similar events take place in renal tubular cells.

Fortunately, most paracetamol overdoses in young children involve paediatric formulations which limit the quantity ingested. As a result, clinically important toxicity is uncommon in this age group. Young children may also metabolize paracetamol differently from their elders and in such a way that the risk of hepatotoxicity is reduced.

Features

Typical poisoning

The typical features of untreated paracetamol toxicity with respect to time since ingestion are shown in Table 4.4. The early symptoms are unremarkable. Nausea and vomiting are frequent within a few hours of the overdose and there may be generalized abdominal pain secondary to the effort of retching and liver tenderness. Loss of consciousness is not a feature unless other CNS depressants have been taken. Patients frequently look paler and more miserable and have more protracted nausea and vomiting after reversal of coma resulting from paracetamol/opioid analgesic combinations. These features are due to the opioid rather than paracetamol and usually subside within 24 hours.

Table 4.4 The timetable of severe, untreated paracetamol overdosage

Time from ingestion (hours)	Feature
<12	Vomiting due to drug
12–36	Vomiting secondary to liver damage
24	Right upper quadrant abdominal pain and tenderness
24–72	Risk of hypoglycaemia
72+	Cerebral oedema
72–96	Grade 3 encephalopathy
	Peak abnormalities of liver function tests
96+	Prothrombin time improves
	Grade 4 encephalopathy
	Brainstem coning

Hepatotoxicity   It is unusual for paracetamol-induced hepatotoxicity to be clinically apparent before 12–36 hours. The usual warning signs comprise continuation of vomiting, localization of abdominal pain to the right subcostal area and tenderness over the liver – features which compel some patients to seek medical help comparatively late after paracetamol overdosage. Jaundice does not usually become obvious before the third or fourth day. Plasma alanine and aspartate aminotransferase (ALT and AST) activity may begin to rise as early as 12 hours but peak values are not usually attained until 72–96 hours after the overdose. Aminotransferase activity of up to 10 000 units/l is common and much higher levels are not unusual. Elevation of the alkaline phosphatase is usually minimal. Plasma bilirubin concentrations rise more slowly than the enzymes and seldom exceed 190 μmol/l (10 mg/dl) in survivors. The International Normalised Ratio (INR) or prothrombin time is often abnormal within 24–36 hours (maximum 48–72 hours).

If hepatocellular necrosis is extensive, hepatic failure ensues on about the fourth or fifth day (though occasionally sooner) with impaired consciousness, confusion, hyperventilation, hypoglycaemia and bleeding secondary to coagulation abnormalities. Fatal cases often develop respiratory or Gram-negative infections, cerebral oedema and disseminated intravascular coagulation.

Renal toxicity   Paracetamol causes renal tubular necrosis in the same way as it produces hepatic necrosis, although it is common in hepatic encephalopathy from any cause. Acute renal failure occurs in only a small proportion of patients, usually, but not always, those with severe liver damage and hepatic failure. In these cases, renal angle pain may be present as early as 12–36 hours after ingestion, and is often associated with albuminuria and haematuria. Plasma creatinine concentrations rise more rapidly than the urea when renal failure develops. Rarely, paracetamol-induced renal failure occurs in the absence of serious liver damage.

Electrolyte and metabolic abnormalities   Hyperglycaemia is occasionally found in some jaundiced patients but severe hypoglycaemia (Table 4.4) is much more important. Some degree of metabolic acidosis is commonly present from the outset and hypophosphataemia secondary to renal phosphate loss has been shown to be a dose-related effect.

Other features   Skin rashes, myocardial necrosis and pancreatitis have also been reported. However, elevation of serum amylase levels is to be expected since amylase is normally removed from the circulation by the liver.

Undisclosed overdosage

It is not uncommon for patients who have taken overdoses of paracetamol to hide the fact until hepatotoxicity forces them to present to general medical, surgical and infectious diseases units as unexplained vomiting, abdominal pain or jaundice. A high index of suspicion is required if the true diagnosis is to be made. Plasma ALT activity >5000 u/l is highly suggestive since such levels are seldom attained in viral hepatitis. Unfortunately, by the time paracetamol overdosage is considered, the drug has usually disappeared from the blood and the laboratory is of little value; only the patient can confirm the diagnosis.

Late presentation

The term 'late presentation' is used to identify patients with paracetamol overdosage who, for one reason or another, do not seek medical help during the time period when antidotes are maximally effective. At present, this means presentation more than 15 hours after ingestion. The delay is not necessarily an attempt to conceal the overdose; the relatively minor early symptoms of poisoning are easily tolerated by many but those due to the onset of features of hepatic necrosis are not and commonly force patients to seek help. Not surprisingly, there is a high morbidity and mortality in this group.

Atypical poisoning

Rare cases of atypical paracetamol poisoning have been reported. The features include severe metabolic acidosis, early loss of consciousness (not due to hypoglycaemia or hepatic encephalopathy) and extremely high plasma paracetamol concentrations (usually >800 mg/l).

Identifying patients at risk of liver damage

The amount of paracetamol ingested

There is general agreement that severe liver damage (defined as peak plasma ALT activity exceeding 1 000 u/l) is likely if more than 250 mg paracetamol/kg body weight has been ingested and unlikely if less than 150 mg/kg has been taken. The fatal dose for an adult may be as little as 12 g.

Identifying additional risk due to liver enzyme induction

Patients who regularly take drugs which induce liver microsomal oxidase systems, including carbamazepine, phenytoin, phenobarbitone, primidone and rifampicin, or alcohol in excess of recommended limits, are at risk from lower plasma paracetamol concentrations than others. It is therefore important that they be identified before management decisions are made.

Plasma paracetamol concentrations

The severity of paracetamol overdosage is best assessed from the plasma paracetamol concentration related to the time from ingestion. About 90% of untreated patients whose plasma paracetamol concentrations related to time lie above line A (Fig. 4.1) develop ALT levels

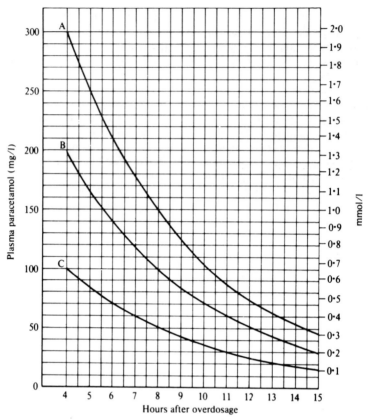

Figure 4.1 Patients whose liver enzymes are not induced and whose plasma paracetamol concentrations related to time from ingestion are above line B require specific treatment as do induced patients above line C

above 1000 units/l and most fatal cases and some of those who develop acute renal failure also come into this group. If all patients above line B are considered, the proportion with plasma ALT above 1000 is about 60% compared with only 25% for those between lines B and C. Line B is the accepted 'treatment' line for those whose liver enzymes are not induced. Line C is the currently recommended treatment line for those whose livers are induced.

In interpreting plasma paracetamol concentrations note:

1 The 'treatment lines' are not infallible. The response of individuals to the same amount of paracetamol is variable and prior consumption of alcohol and other drugs may modify it further.

2 The time interval since ingestion is critical and often difficult to establish. Obtaining the best estimate requires more effort in detailed questioning than some doctors seem prepared to make.

3 Plasma concentrations taken within 4 hours of ingestion cannot reliably be interpreted because the drug is still being absorbed and distributed.

4 The validity of line B beyond 15 hours is uncertain because of the paucity of data from untreated patients. However, patients who present late tend to be more severely poisoned and at greater risk of serious liver damage. Poisons information centres may be able to advise on the significance of late plasma paracetamol concentrations.

5 Treatment line B was developed from observation in adults. No studies have been carried out to ascertain its appropriateness to young children and ethical considerations probably now prohibit them.

6 One has no choice but to assume that the time–plasma paracetamol liver damage relationship applies equally to poisoning with paracetamol/opioid analgesic combinations but it should be remembered that the latter delay gastric emptying. Higher plasma concentrations are therefore obtained later than they would have been had paracetamol been taken alone. Patients who have late high plasma concentrations after overdosage with opioid-containing formulations do not seem to develop liver damage as frequently as might be expected.

Antidotes

It has been shown clinically and experimentally that paracetamol-induced liver damage, renal failure and death can be prevented by the administration of sulphydryl donors such as methionine and N-acetylcysteine. They act as precursors of glutathione.

N-acetylcysteine
Actions. When given in the early stages of poisoning, N-acetylcysteine acts as a glutathione precursor while after 24 hours or more any benefit is probably due to other actions including that of a free radical scavenger. It provides virtually complete protection against liver damage when given to those at risk within 8 hours of the overdose but its efficacy declines thereafter. However, there is still considerable protection up to 10 hours and even from 10 to 12 hours. Early trials suggested that it was ineffective when given later than 15 hours after ingestion and there was concern that it might predispose to the development of hepatic encephalopathy. Its use beyond that time was therefore considered contraindicated. However, several years of experience indicate that there is no additional risk in giving acetylcysteine late

Table 4.5 N-acetylcysteine doses for intravenous injection

Dose	N-acetylcysteine (mg/kg body weight)	Volume of 5% dextrose for dilution	Duration of infusion
1	150	200 ml	15 min
2	50	500 ml	4 hours
3	50	500 ml	8 hours
4	50	500 ml	8 hours

and that it is tolerated well, even by patients who have fulminant hepatic necrosis. There is now, therefore, no time limit on its administration and controlled studies indicate that late treatment reduces morbidity and mortality.

Dosage and routes of administration. In the UK, acetylcysteine is given intravenously according to the dosage schedule given in Table 4.5. Oral N-acetylcysteine (140 mg/kg body weight followed by 70 mg/kg 4 hourly for 17 doses) is used in the USA although a 48-hour intravenous regimen has recently been described.

Adverse effects. The frequency of adverse effects from N-acetylcysteine has varied considerably from one study to another, the highest estimate being about 15%. The features have been described as anaphylactoid but are very similar to those of dose-related toxicity. They are most common in the first hour of treatment, a relatively short time during which more than half of the total dose to be given over 20 hours has been infused. Nausea, flushing, urticaria and pruritus are amongst the most common while angioedema, wheezing, respiratory distress, hypotension and hypertension are fortunately rare. Occasionally, skin reactions are limited to the area of the infusion site. Their management is usually simple. Minor reactions often clear rapidly with stopping the infusion for a short time and without additional measures. It should then be possible to re-start the infusion at the lowest rate (100 mg/kg body weight over 16 hours). Should more serious features develop, stop the infusion and give an antihistamine. Corticosteroids should seldom be necessary.

Methionine
Oral methionine (2.5 g 4-hourly to a total of 10 g) is advocated by some centres but in one study 10% of patients treated in this way subsequently had AST levels above 1000 units/l. Methionine has no significant adverse effects.

Which antidote?
The choice of antidote for the prophylaxis of severe liver damage after paracetamol overdosage is dictated by national availability, the

occurrence of vomiting, the time since ingestion and geographical considerations. In the UK, the choice lies between intravenous *N*-acetylcysteine and oral methionine. The latter is considerably less expensive than the former but, since it has to be given orally, is inappropriate for patients who are vomiting. The incidence of vomiting after paracetamol overdosage seems to vary from one part of the country to another but few would argue that it is very common in the patients at highest risk of liver damage. *N*-acetylcysteine is therefore the treatment of choice for the latter. However, methionine has an important role in the management of paracetamol poisoning in geographically remote areas where intravenous antidotes may neither be available nor practicable. At-risk patients who present longer than 10 hours after ingestion should receive acetylcysteine since there is no evidence that methionine is of value at this stage.

Management of overdosage in young children

Few young children will require active treatment after accidental paracetamol overdosage. If they do, there is no choice but to manage them as adults.

Management of older children and adults at specific ingestion/presentation intervals

The clinician managing paracetamol overdosage has to decide whether or not to empty the stomach, identify the patients at risk of developing severe liver damage taking appropriate cognisance of possible liver enzyme induction (see above), decide which of the latter should be treated with antidotes and institute treatment with appropriate urgency.

Presentation within 4 hours of ingestion
1 Empty the stomach if more than 150 mg/kg has been taken within 4 hours.
2 Give activated charcoal.
3 Wait until 4 hours have elapsed since ingestion before taking blood for urgent estimation of the plasma paracetamol concentration.
4 Give a dose of methionine orally if more than 150 mg paracetamol/kg has been taken and there will be a delay before blood for the plasma paracetamol concentration can be taken.
5 Consider whether or not the patient's liver enzymes are induced (see above).
6 Assess the risk of the patient developing severe liver damage by considering the plasma paracetamol concentration related to the time from ingestion, as shown in Figure 4.1.

7 Give an antidote immediately to patients whose paracetamol concentrations related to time from ingestion lie above the relevant treatment line in Figure 4.1.
8 Determine the INR and plasma creatinine concentration at the end of N-acetylcysteine infusion and before discharging the patient.
9 Provided the antidote is started within 8 hours of ingestion, patients may be discharged on completion of its administration. Protection should be complete after such early treatment and there is no merit in keeping them in hospital simply to measure serial liver function tests. In the unusual circumstance that protection has been less than complete, there is no specific treatment and patients can be advised to return if vomiting or abdominal pain recurs.

Presentation 4–8 hours after ingestion
1 It is too late for gastric emptying and activated charcoal to be of value.
2 Take blood immediately for urgent estimation of the plasma paracetamol concentration.
3 Management is then identical to that given for presentation within 4 hours.

Presentation 8–15 hours after ingestion
Presentation at this interval after ingestion calls for prompt and empiric action which inevitably results in the unnecessary treatment of some patients but is justified by the need to minimize hepatic damage (with a possibly fatal outcome) in those at risk and the low incidence of serious adverse effects from N-acetylcysteine.

1 Speed is of the essence. The efficacy of antidotes is declining rapidly at this time after ingestion.
2 Give N-acetylcysteine immediately without waiting for the plasma paracetamol concentration if more than 150 mg/kg or a total of 12 g has been ingested.
3 Take blood for estimation of the plasma paracetamol concentration and use the result in the usual way to assess the risk of the patient developing severe liver damage. Be sure to use line C (Figure 4.1) for those whose liver enzymes may be induced.
4 Stop administration of the antidote if assessment indicates that the likelihood of liver damage is low.
5 Continue administration of the antidote if assessment indicates a risk of severe liver damage.
6 Determine the INR and plasma creatinine concentration at the end of N-acetylcysteine infusion.

7 Patients who are asymptomatic and do not have significant prolongation of INR or elevation of plasma creatinine may be discharged.
8 Monitor patients who have symptoms or laboratory evidence of liver and/or renal damage.

Presentation 15–24 hours after ingestion
Patients who present 15 hours or longer after overdosage usually do so because they have developed intolerable symptoms. Clinical impression suggests that they are at much greater risk of developing serious liver necrosis.

1 Give *N*-acetylcysteine immediately to every case.
2 Take blood on admission for determination of the plasma paracetamol concentration, INR and plasma creatinine concentration.
3 Stop treating and discharge patients who are asymptomatic, and in whom the INR and plasma creatinine are normal and the plasma paracetamol concentration is less than 10 mg/l (0.07 mmol/l) 24 hours or less after ingestion.
4 Monitor patients who have symptoms or laboratory evidence of liver and/or renal damage.

Presentation more than 24 hours after ingestion
The appropriate management of this group of patients with paracetamol overdosage is still a matter for debate. Further studies are required to determine the value of *N*-acetylcysteine at this time after overdosage and may be available soon. To obtain the most up-to-date views on the management of late cases, it is therefore important to contact a poisons information centre once the patient's INR, plasma creatinine concentration and arterial hydrogen ion concentration are known.

Supportive measures
Vitamin K_1 should be given though it is unlikely to be effective. Administration of fresh frozen plasma or clotting factor concentrates should be reserved for the treatment of active haemorrhage. Avoid administration of CNS depressant drugs if at all possible and monitor blood glucose concentrations. The patient should be regularly screened for evidence of infection and renal failure. The best guides to renal function are the urine output and plasma creatinine. The plasma urea may not rise until relatively late since urea production is diminished by extensive hepatic necrosis. Careful control of fluid and electrolyte balance is essential. Haemodialysis may be required for renal failure. Correction of hypophosphataemia is important.
    Assisted ventilation can be instituted at an early stage in the hope of delaying the onset and severity of cerebral oedema and mannitol and

haemofiltration may also be helpful. The coagulation disturbance may preclude intracranial pressure monitoring

Liver transplantation

Liver transplantation is now a feasible option for some patients with fulminant hepatic failure secondary to paracetamol overdosage. The problem is to identify them at a sufficiently early stage that they can be transferred as safely as possible to appropriate centres and to allow time for assessment by the transplant team, find a donor organ and complete the operation. Inevitably, only a fraction of such patients will ultimately have a transplant. Current knowledge suggests that patients who are acidaemic, hypotensive (mean systolic blood pressure <60 mmHg), encephalopathic or are known to have pre-existing liver disease should be considered possible candidates for liver transplantation.

Possible contraindications should be clarified by discussion but currently include:

1 Infection which has been treated for less than 48 hours.
2 Inability to raise the systolic blood pressure above 90 mmHg, even using inotropes.
3 Cerebral oedema with impaired brainstem function.
4 A clear and repeated wish to die expressed before the onset of encephalopathy.
5 A history of repeated episodes of parasuicide.

Common special circumstances

Unexpectedly high plasma concentrations

It is not uncommon to encounter patients whose plasma paracetamol concentrations seem unusually high for the time after ingestion (i.e. they are well above line B in Fig. 4.1). The most likely explanation is that the time interval has been overestimated. Alternatively, absorption may have been delayed by some other drug taken concomitantly. They must be given N-acetylcysteine immediately but may not be at as much risk as first seems.

The two-stage overdose

Some patients, disillusioned by the lack of effects from one overdose of paracetamol, take a second within a few hours. Clearly, this creates difficulty in assessing the risk of liver damage and the need for antidotes. The only solution is to interpret the plasma paracetamol concentration as if were the result of all the drug having been ingested at time of the first overdose. This overestimates the potential seriousness of the situation but errs on the safe side and is justified by the safety of treatment.

Overdosage during pregnancy

Paracetamol overdosage during pregnancy is not uncommon. The health of the mother must take priority and she should be assessed and treated as any other patient. While maternal overdosage can lead to fetal liver damage and intrauterine death, the now considerable evidence which is available suggests that abortions and teratogenic effects are uncommon. Paracetamol overdosage, alone, is therefore not an indication for termination of pregnancy or premature delivery. Nor does treatment with antidotes appear to carry any risk to the fetus.

Prognosis

The mortality from paracetamol poisoning is very low but the number of deaths is increasing as the drug is used ever more widely for self-poisoning. If deaths are to be avoided, doctors must be aware of its dangers in overdosage, that an effective antidote is available and, above all, that effective treatment is a matter of great urgency. The greater the degree of acidosis on presentation and the faster the PT lengthens, the more likely is a fatal outcome. Patients who present with an arterial hydrogen ion concentration of >50 nmol/l (pH <7.3), have a peak PT of >180 seconds or whose PT increases between the third and fourth day after ingestion have a greater than 90% chance of dying. Most deaths are due to cerebral oedema complicating fulminant hepatic failure and occur in patients who present late. The fortunate aspect of paracetamol overdosage is that patients who recover from even severe hepatic necrosis regain normal liver histology without evidence of cirrhosis. Reports of long-term complications are rare. Likewise, recovery of renal function should be complete.

References

Bray GP, Mowat C, Muir DF *et al.* The effect of chronic alcohol intake on prognosis and outcome in paracetamol overdose. *Hum Exp Toxicol* 1991; **10**: 435–438.

Davenport A, Finn R. Paracetamol (acetaminophen) poisoning resulting in acute renal failure without hepatic coma. *Nephron* 1988; **50**: 55–56.

Dawson AH, Henry DA, McEwen J. Adverse reactions to *N*-acetylcysteine during treatment for paracetamol poisoning. *Med J Aust* 1989; **150**: 329–331.

Flanagan RJ, Meredith TJ. Use of *N*-acetylcysteine in clinical toxicology. *Am J Med* 1991; **91** (Suppl 3C): 3C-131S–3C-139S.

Jones AF, Harvey JM, Vale JA. Hypophosphataemia and phosphaturia in paracetamol poisoning. *Lancet* 1989; **ii**: 608–609.

Keays R, Harrison PM, Wendon JA *et al.* Intravenous acetylcysteine in paracetamol induced fulminant hepatic failure: a controlled trial. *Br Med J* 1991; **303**: 1026–1029.

McElhatton PR, Sullivan FM, Volans GN *et al.* Paracetamol poisoning in pregnancy: an analysis of the outcome of cases referred to the Teratology Information Service of the National Poisons Information Service. *Hum Exp Toxicol* 1990; **9**: 147–153.

Meredith TJ, Prescott LF, Vale JA. Why do patients still die from paracetamol poisoning? *Br Med J* 1986; **293**: 345–346.

O'Grady JG, Wendon J, Tan KC *et al.* Liver transplantation after paracetamol overdose. *Br Med J* 1991; **303**: 221–223.

Parker D, White JP, Paton D *et al.* Safety of late acetylcysteine treatment in paracetamol poisoning. *Hum Exp Toxicol* 1990; **2**: 25–27.

Penna A, Buchanan N. Paracetamol poisoning in children and hepatotoxicity. *Br J Clin Pharmacol* 1991; **32**: 143–149.

Prescott LF, Donovan JW, Jarvie DR *et al.* The disposition and kinetics of intravenous acetylcysteine in patients with paracetamol poisoning. *Eur J Clin Pharmacol* 1989; **37**: 501–506.

Riggs BS, Bronstein AC, Kulig K *et al.* Acute acetaminophen overdose during pregnancy. *Obstet Gynecol* 1989; **74**: 247–253.

Smilkstein MJ, Bronstein AC, Linden C *et al.* Acetaminophen overdose: a 48-hour intravenous *N*-acetylcysteine treatment protocol. *Ann Emerg Med* 1991; **20**: 1058–1063.

Wakeel RA, Davis HT, Williams JD. Toxic myocarditis in paracetamol poisoning. *Br Med J* 1987; **295**: 1097.

Paraquat

General considerations

Paraquat is a bipyridilium herbicide which attracted much concern following a number of deaths from accidental ingestion of what appeared to be very small quantities of the 20% solution, Gramoxone, in the late 1960s. The high mortality, the publicity surrounding its subsequent use for homicide and the belief that little could be done to influence the course of poisoning added to its notoriety. Fortunately, accidental paraquat poisoning in the UK has become uncommon and, happily, the number of occasions on which it is used for self-poisoning is also considerably less than it was formerly. Self-poisoning now accounts for most cases and paraquat remains a common means of committing suicide, particularly in Japan and Sri Lanka. Though paraquat poisoning is the mode of death for a substantial number of suicides throughout the world, proper use produces incalculable benefits by improving agricultural productivity in developing countries where it is used extensively. Some products and their contents are shown in Table 4.6.

Only about 5% of ingested paraquat is absorbed but absorption is rapid, the volume of distribution high and there is evidence of energy-dependent accumulation in some organs, particularly lung. Faecal excretion of paraquat continues for many days, suggesting the possibility of enterohepatic circulation of the poison. While some absorbed paraquat may be eliminated in the faeces, most is excreted in the urine, possibly by tubular secretion.

Table 4.6 Liquid and granular products containing paraquat

Product	Formulation	Paraquat ion content	Other ingredients
Cleansweep	Liquid	100 g/l	Diquat
Dexuron	Liquid	100 g/l	Diuron
Farmon PDQ	Liquid	120 g/l	Diquat
Gramazine	Liquid	100 g/l	Simazine
Gramonol	Liquid	100 g/l	Monolinuron
Gramonol 5	Liquid	110 g/l	Monolinuron
Gramonol Five	Liquid	110 g/l	Monolinuron
Gramoxone 100	Liquid	200 g/l	
Groundhog	Granules	25 g/kg	Amitrole, diquat, simazine
Pathclear	Granules	25 g/kg	Amitrole, diquat, simazine
Scythe	Liquid	200 g/l	
Terraklene	Liquid	100 g/l	Simazine
Tota-col	Liquid	100 g/l	Diuron
Weedol	Granules	25 g/kg	Diquat

Sufficient paraquat can be absorbed percutaneously to cause serious and fatal systemic poisoning but this is very uncommon. In contrast, serious poisoning has not been reported after inhalation of sprayed solutions containing paraquat.

Solutions of paraquat are corrosive and it is a multiorgan poison which has its most unique and lethal effects on the lungs, producing histological and functional changes similar to those of oxygen poisoning. Animal experiments have shown that the pulmonary toxicity is increased by high inspired oxygen tensions, supporting the suggestion that the toxicity of paraquat is due to the formation of superoxide radicals.

Features

The features of paraquat poisoning depend on the route and magnitude of exposure and a small number of scenarios recur frequently.

Inhalation of spray
Inhalation of spray of dilute paraquat solutions often occurs in windy weather and when face masks are not being worn. Fortunately the consequences are seldom serious. A sore throat, husky voice and, in some cases, epistaxis, are usually all that develops.

Skin contamination
Leakage from spray canisters carried on the back has caused skin ulceration and a few patients have developed features of systemic

poisoning (as detailed below). Deaths have been reported from this type of accident but skin splashes which are promptly and thoroughly dealt with should not occasion fear of systemic toxicity.

Splashes in the eyes

Paraquat in the eyes causes intense spasm of the eyelids, lacrimation, and corneal ulceration.

Ingestion of recently sprayed crops

Occasionally, crops which have been recently contaminated with diluted paraquat are eaten. It is highly improbable that any individual could consume a sufficient quantity of the vegetable to be at risk provided the herbicide was correctly diluted before use. Should there be any doubt about the magnitude of exposure, urine and blood paraquat concentrations can be checked as below.

Ingestion of large amounts

Potentially lethal poisoning occurs most commonly after deliberate ingestion of 1.5 g or more of paraquat, the amount contained in one sachet of Weedol or a small mouthful of Gramoxone. Paraquat has four major effects including corrosion of the gastrointestinal tract, hepatic necrosis, renal tubular necrosis and a complex sequence of pulmonary abnormalities culminating in progressive intra-alveolar fibrosis. The severity of these lesions and the speed with which each develops depends largely on the quantity of paraquat ingested. Three common clinical courses can be identified.

The most rapid course follows ingestion of 6 g or more of paraquat. Nausea, vomiting, abdominal pain and diarrhoea occur within an hour or so and the patient becomes cold, clammy and hypotensive, partly due to fluid loss and partly as the result of myocardial depression. A metabolic acidosis is frequently present, consciousness may be impaired and convulsions may occur. Within 12–24 hours there is increasing breathlessness and cyanosis due to acute chemical-induced pulmonary oedema. Death follows quickly before buccal ulceration and hepatic and renal necrosis become problems. At autopsy the lungs are found to be oedematous and haemorrhagic.

The second course is more protracted and follows ingestion of 3–6 g of paraquat. The early signs of gastrointestinal irritation are present but shock does not develop. The alimentary features usually subside within 24 hours, by which time pain in the mouth and throat becomes prominent making it difficult to swallow, speak or cough. The mucous membranes of the lips, mouth and tongue become white in colour before desquamating patchily to leave painful red, raw surfaces after about 3 days. Dysphagia due to such lesions may compel patients who conceal ingestion of paraquat to present to hospital, often at ear, nose and throat departments. Perforation of the oesophagus with subsequent mediastinitis has been reported and some patients have vomited pieces of oesophageal and gastric mucosa. Others have been found to have the oesophageal lining coiled in the stomach at autopsy. Laboratory evidence of hepatocellular and renal tubular necrosis is usually obvious by about 72 hours but jaundice is seldom severe unless the patient has preexisting liver disease. In contrast, renal damage is usually severe and may require treatment by haemodialysis. Breathlessness, tachypnoea, widespread crepitations and central cyanosis may be present by 5–7 days after ingestion and progress relentlessly until the patient dies from hypoxia a few days later. In such cases the lungs show alveolar oedema containing fibroblasts but haemorrhage tends to be less obvious than in patients dying earlier.

The slowest course may follow ingestion of 1.5–2.0 g of paraquat (the contents of a sachet of Weedol). Nausea, vomiting and diarrhoea occur and renal tubular damage is usual but tends to be mild. Liver damage of any consequence is uncommon. Complaints of pain in the throat occur frequently but frank ulceration is unusual. Respiratory involvement may not be apparent till 10–21 days after ingestion. Breathlessness, basal crepitations and bilateral chest X-ray opacities are the earliest signs and progress till the patient dies as late as 5 or 6 weeks after taking the paraquat, by which time the local corrosive effects and hepatic and renal necrosis have resolved. The lungs are found to be excessively heavy and rubbery as is consistent with extensive intra- and interalveolar fibrosis shown histologically.

Poisoning in pregnancy
Ingestion of large amounts of paraquat during pregnancy is likely to cause fetal death whether or not emergency caesarean section is performed.

Screening tests for paraquat

Urine
Detection of paraquat in the urine is a simple matter particularly if the urine has been voided within a few hours of ingestion. Urine (5 ml) is made alkaline by adding sufficient sodium bicarbonate to cover the point of a knife followed by a similar quantity of sodium dithionite. If paraquat is present a blue colour develops immediately, the depth of colour increasing with the concentration of paraquat. A pale green colour may be obtained with diquat or low concentrations of paraquat.

The absorption and initial renal excretion of paraquat are so rapid that failure to obtain a positive test on urine passed within 4 hours of alleged ingestion can be interpreted as indicating that no significant quantity of paraquat has been absorbed. This simple test is therefore of great value in accidental exposure, e.g. inhalation or ingestion of very small quantities.

Plasma
High plasma concentrations can be crudely anticipated in the ward sideroom by applying the urine screening test to 2–3 ml of plasma. The darker the blue colour which develops, the higher the plasma concentration. A faint blue colour is given with 2–4 mg/l.

Management of skin and eye contamination

Eye contamination is managed as described on p. 109. Skin ulcers without systemic toxicity are treated as burns.

Management of poisoning by ingestion

There is no evidence that the outcome of paraquat poisoning can be altered by medical intervention. Therapeutic gloom has prevailed for years, relieved only occasionally and transiently by reports of success in animal studies or uncontrolled (usually solitary) human observations. There has been no lack of effort; corticosteroids, drugs to prevent free radical formation, free radical scavengers, immunosuppressive agents, whole-bowel irrigation, haemodialysis, haemoperfusion, radiotherapy to the lungs and lung transplantation have all been tried without convincing evidence that they have reduced mortality. The reason is simple. On the one hand, time for intervention is at a premium with this toxin since potentially lethal amounts can be absorbed within as little as an hour of ingestion and, on the other, it takes too long to institute the measures which might have a beneficial effect. Adsorbents are not normally available at the scenes of incidents and the elimination techniques that might have an impact are available only at selected centres and take too long to initiate. Even if the latter could be overcome there would still be good reasons for lack of efficacy; plasma concentrations of paraquat are low, they decline very rapidly and currently available techniques are far from sufficiently efficient.

Preventing absorption
The only intervention of possible value is to give an adsorbent as a matter of the greatest urgency in the hope of binding paraquat in the stomach and thereby preventing further absorption. Fuller's earth

(200 ml of a 30% aqueous solution), bentonite (200 ml of a 7% suspension in water and glycerine) or activated charcoal will do. All of them bind paraquat strongly. Repeated doses may be given but are of doubtful merit and one should not persist with them to the point of adding to patient distress.

Although it is traditional to empty the stomach despite the corrosive effects of the poison, it is doubtful if it is of any value by the time it is done. Adsorbents are much more efficient.

Whole-bowel irrigation may facilitate paraquat absorption unless a binding agent is added to the irrigation fluid.

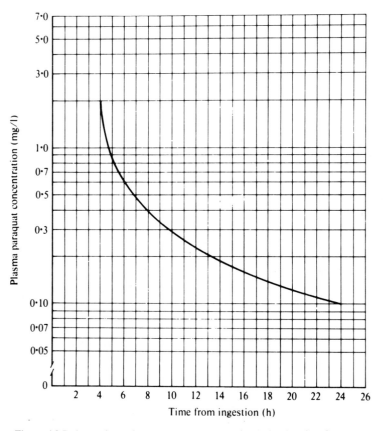

Figure 4.2 Patients whose plasma paraquat concentrations related to time from ingestion are above the line are likely to die, and those below survive. There are insufficient data to interpret concentrations measured within 4 hours

Elimination techniques
Forced diuresis and peritoneal dialysis are of no value and the available evidence indicates that neither haemodialysis nor charcoal haemoperfusion can rapidly remove toxicologically significant quantities of paraquat. Despite this, the latter has been recommended for patients with plasma paraquat concentrations close to the prognostic line (Fig 4.2) in the hope that the elimination of even very small quantities will tip the balance in favour of survival. In reality, few patients in this group receive such treatment. If it is done, the very low plasma paraquat concentrations would make charcoal haemoperfusion preferable to haemodialysis, and it must be started as early as possible and continued as intensively as practicable during the first 24–48 hours. The decision as to when to stop should be guided by plasma paraquat measurements.

Symptomatic measures
Antiemetics and analgesics will be required in some cases and intravenous fluids may be necessary to replace gastrointestinal losses. Mouth and laryngeal burns may be extremely painful and require considerable nursing care. Patients who are likely to die should be kept as comfortable as possible.

Prognosis

The mortality from ingestion of any quantity of Gramoxone is about 60% and with Weedol (about a sachet or more) is about 10%. Perhaps the most ominous feature is the onset of renal failure which effectively prevents the elimination of absorbed paraquat. Few patients survive paraquat lung damage.

Since peak plasma concentrations of paraquat are usually achieved within 4 hours, before most patients arrive at hospital, it seems that the outcome is already determined.

The prognosis in individual cases can be predicted from the plasma paraquat concentration related to the time from ingestion. Patients whose levels fall below the line (Fig 4.2) will almost certainly survive without treatment while those with levels well above the line are extremely likely to die regardless of what is done for them. Any patient whose plasma paraquat concentration exceeds 0.1 mg/l after 25 hours is unlikely to survive. However, since there is no effective treatment, it is doubtful if quantitative assay on an urgent basis can be justified; analysis on the first 'working' day is probably sufficient. Early assessment of prognosis facilitates the management of patients and their relatives.

References

Franzen D, Mecking H, Kaferatein H *et al*. Failure of radiotherapy to resolve fatal lung damage due to paraquat poisoning. *Chest* 1990; **100**: 1164–1165.

Hoffer E, Taitelman U. Exposure to paraquat through skin absorption: clinical and laboratory observations of accidental splashing on healthy skin of agricultural workers. *Hum Toxicol* 1989; **8**: 483–485.

Houze P, Baud FJ, Mouy R *et al*. Toxicokinetics of paraquat in humans. *Hum Exp Toxicol* 1990; **9**: 5–12.

Ikebuchi J. Evaluation of paraquat concentrations in paraquat poisoning. *Arch Toxicol* 1987; **60**: 304–310.

Pond SM. Manifestations and management of paraquat poisoning. *Med J Aust* 1990; **152**: 256–259.

Talbot AR, Fu CC. Paraquat intoxication during pregnancy: a report of 9 cases. *Vet Hum Toxicol* 1988; **30**: 12–17.

Petroleum distillates and turpentine

Diesel fuel	Naphtha
Furniture polishes	Paraffin
Gasoline	Petrol
Kerosene	Turpentine
Lighter fluid	Turpentine substitute

General considerations

Petroleum distillates and turpentine are considered together because they have similar toxicological effects although they are chemically different. The term petroleum distillates refers to a group of solvents and fuels which contain differing proportions of a wide variety of aliphatic and aromatic hydrocarbons. Turpentine comprises a mixture of pinenes, camphenes and other terpenes and should not be confused with turpentine substitute (white spirit), a mixture of long chain hydro-carbons which is extensively used as a paint thinner.

Ingestion of petroleum distillates is a common childhood problem because they are readily available in most households, including developing countries where kerosene, in particular, is used for heating, cooking and lighting. In both affluent and developing societies petroleum distillates are frequently kept in inappropriate, unlabelled containers thereby increasing the likelihood of accidental childhood poisoning.

Adults may deliberately ingest large quantities but are perhaps more likely to be poisoned accidentally in the course of siphoning petrol or gasoline from car fuel tanks. Petroleum distillates are also used as solvents for some pesticides and may add to their toxicity when ingested or inhaled.

Though ingestion is by far the commonest route for poisoning, absorption of petroleum distillates by inhalation is also possible (see volatile substance abuse, p. 223). Deliberate self-injection with these compounds has rarely been reported and systemic poisoning has followed the use of diesel fuel as a shampoo and for repeated hand-washing.

Features

Ingestion of petroleum distillates usually produces remarkably little upset. Vomiting is common but by no means invariable while diarrhoea is uncommon. Cerebral function is usually altered with some patients becoming excited and agitated but more often there is drowsiness leading (in severe poisoning) to coma. Convulsions occur rarely.

Most concern about petroleum distillate poisoning has centred on the pulmonary complications which occur in up to 60% of cases and result from aspiration into the bronchial tree rather than from blood-borne hydrocarbon absorbed from the gastrointestinal tract. However, the higher blood concentrations attained by intravenous injection of these compounds may produce the same pulmonary changes as aspiration. The high incidence of respiratory complications in patients who do not vomit may be explained by the rapidity and ease with which some hydrocarbons with low surface tensions spread over large areas.

Clinical and radiological evidence of lung involvement is often apparent within minutes but in some cases may be delayed for up to 24 hours. Cough, choking, wheezing and breathlessness are the main symptoms and the smell of the hydrocarbon is usually detectable on the breath. Central cyanosis may be present but auscultation of the lungs is often unrewarding, even in patients with respiratory distress. Severe poisoning causes haemorrhagic pulmonary oedema which is fatal within 24 hours. Radiologically the pneumonitis usually involves two or more lobes and is occasionally perihilar in distribution.

Fever and a polymorph leucocytosis are common, even in the absence of a pneumonitis. Rare complications include pneumatocele formation, intravascular haemolysis and renal failure.

Diagnosis of hydrocarbon ingestion may be confirmed by finding a double gastric fluid level on an X-ray of the abdomen taken in the erect posture. This is produced by the layer of hydrocarbon floating between the gastric juice and the air bubble.

Management

The question of whether the stomach should be emptied after ingestion of petroleum distillates has been the centre of controversy for many years. While the traditional assumption that induced vomiting and gastric lavage increase the incidence of hydrocarbon pneumonitis has been refuted by the majority of recent studies, there is equally no good evidence that they are of any benefit. Nevertheless, because of the risk of severe toxicity or the development of rare complications, present-day opinion favours emptying the stomach if a large amount has been ingested and provided the patient is sufficiently alert to be able to cough effectively or the airway can be protected by insertion of a cuffed endotracheal tube. The following are regarded as indications for gastric emptying:

1 Ingestion of >1 ml/kg body weight (assuming a 'mouthful' in a 2- or 3-year-old child to be of the order of 4–5 ml).
2 The solution contains another toxin (e.g. a pesticide).
3 Signs of serious poisoning are already present.

Administration of olive oil reduces the absorption of petroleum distillates but unfortunately increases the incidence of pneumonitis and is not recommended.

Clinical and laboratory studies have failed to show any benefit from corticosteroids and routine antibiotics in patients with respiratory complications. Antibiotics should be reserved for those who develop proven secondary bacterial infection.

Oxygen may be necessary if cyanosis is present and intermittent positive pressure respiration should be considered for patients with pulmonary oedema.

Prognosis

The mortality from ingestion of petroleum distillates is considerably less than 1% and death is invariably the result of hydrocarbon pneumonitis. The latter usually reaches its peak within 24 hours of onset and settles 3–4 days later. There are no reports of long-term lung damage.

Reference

Truemper E, de la Rocha SR, Atkinson SD. Clinical characteristics, pathophysiology, and management of hydrocarbon ingestion: case report and review of the literature. *Pediatr Emerg Care* 1987; **3**: 187–193.

Phencyclidine

General considerations

Phencyclidine was originally developed as an intravenous anaesthetic for human use but was abandoned because of an unacceptably high incidence of postoperative psychotic reactions. It is comparatively easy

to synthesize, being considerably less expensive than other hallucino-
gens such as LSD. Phencyclidine has become a major drug of abuse in
North America and elsewhere. It is often sold to unwitting buyers as
THC or LSD. Although liquid and tablet formulations exist, oral and
intravenous use is uncommon. Phencyclidine is most commonly
available as a white crystal-like powder which is smoked after mixing
with tobacco or some variety of cannabis. Even among users it has a
reputation for causing 'bad trips' and other side-effects.

Features

The clinical features of phencyclidine intoxication are dose-related. If
smoked it produces euphoria, perceptual distortion, numbness and
paraesthesiae, staggering and somewhat drunken behaviour. With
higher doses, however, anxiety and agitation become prominent features
together with hallucinations and muscle rigidity which makes walking
slow and stiff. The pulse rate and systolic and diastolic blood pressures
are commonly raised and hyperventilation and increased oropharyngeal
secretions occur frequently. The individual may alternate between
sitting rigidly with staring eyes and unpredictable violence. Deaths are
most likely to occur during this phase of disturbed behaviour, drowning
being particularly common. With increasing doses and particularly oral
use, muscle twitching, facial grimacing, torticollis, convulsions and
opisthotonus occur until coma, respiratory failure and paralysis
supervene. Rhabdomyolysis has been reported after intravenous and
oral administration. Tolerance and psychological dependence develop
but an abstinence syndrome has not been described.

Discontinuation of phencyclidine may be followed by irritability,
depression and impaired memory lasting several months.

Management

The stomach should be emptied if the drug has been ingested within the
preceding 2 hours. Patients who are hyperexcitable should be stimulated
as little as possible to minimize the risk of violent outbursts. Some,
however, may require physical restraint till they can be adequately
sedated. Haloperidol has been recommended but adequate doses of
diazepam may be just as useful and also have the advantage of
preventing convulsions. Severe tachycardia and hypertension may be
controlled by propranolol. Unconscious patients require the usual
supportive measures with particular attention to gentle removal of
excessive secretions.

Urinary elimination of phencyclidine can be increased by inducing an
acid diuresis but this is no longer used. Disturbed behaviour can be
expected during the recovery phase.

Reference

Leikin JB, Krantz AJ, Zell-Kanter M *et al*. Clinical features and management of intoxication due to hallucinogenic drugs. *Med Toxicol Adv Drug Exp* 1989; **4**: 324–350.

Phenobarbitone

General considerations

Serious poisoning with phenobarbitone is uncommon. Most patients who deliberately poison themselves with this drug are epileptics or close relatives of epileptics. Phenobarbitone poisoning is considered separate from poisoning by barbiturate hypnotics because its features and treatment differ sufficiently to warrant special mention.

Features

The dominant features of acute phenobarbitone intoxication are those of CNS depression but coma, if present, is seldom deeper than grade 2 or grade 3. It is unusual for patients poisoned with this drug to require endotracheal intubation or assisted ventilation and serious hypotension and hypothermia are uncommon. However the long plasma half-life of phenobarbitone (of the order of 3 days) makes recovery slow and symptoms persist for many days. Patients who are not unconscious remain drowsy, dysarthric and ataxic with gross, coarse nystagmus on the slightest movement of the eyes. Their management is made particularly difficult by their disinhibited mental state. They are frequently demanding, argumentative, loquacious, truculent and oblivious to reason. They repeatedly insist on leaving when they are clearly very much under the influence of the drug and a potential danger to themselves and others. More than most patients recovering from drug overdosage, they are very likely to disrupt the normal functioning of medical units for several days.

Plasma phenobarbitone concentrations

Plasma phenobarbitone concentrations of up to 300–400 mg/l may be encountered in acute poisoning but they correlate poorly with clinical severity, partly as a result of tolerance in patients (usually epileptics) already on long-term treatment. Plasma concentrations frequently continue to rise in the first 48 hours after ingestion, during which time the patient may be improving clinically.

Consciousness with disinhibited behaviour is common with plasma phenobarbitone concentrations up to 100 mg/l or occasionally as high as 150 mg/l.

Management

Patients who are unconscious should be given supportive care. Repeated doses of oral activated charcoal greatly shorten the half-life of phenobarbitone and should be given until consciousness is regained. Charcoal has replaced forced alkaline diuresis as the treatment of choice and should also render more intensive elimination techniques such as haemoperfusion unnecessary. Emergency measurement of the plasma phenobarbitone concentration is of no value except in very severe poisoning when invasive measures to increase elimination of the drug are being considered. Assessment of clinical progress will usually make daily measurements of phenobarbitone concentrations superfluous.

Patients in grade 4 coma, those in other grades who develop serious complications and those who are not responding satisfactorily to repeated oral charcoal should be considered for treatment by haemodialysis or charcoal haemoperfusion provided the plasma drug concentrations are sufficiently high (p. 51). Charcoal haemoperfusion removes phenobarbitone more efficiently than haemodialysis.

The management of patients with behavioural disturbances due to phenobarbitone is difficult and may be dictated as much by the other responsibilities of the medical and nursing team at the time as by the needs of the poisoned patient. Sedation with chlorpromazine (50–100 mg intramuscularly) is usually effective and may be required while other measures are undertaken to ensure rapid elimination of the phenobarbitone. However, the patient may not accept this and sedating patients against their wishes raises difficult ethical problems. Such patients place a tremendous strain on the patience and good humour of the nursing staff who carry the brunt of placating and cajoling them into cooperating.

Prognosis

The vast majority of patients poisoned with phenobarbitone who reach hospital recover within a few days with supportive care and repeated doses of oral charcoal. However, in severe poisoning coma may last several days and the risks of life-threatening respiratory infection are considerable, particularly if endotracheal intubation or assisted ventilation is required. Survival in these cases depends on energetic measures to remove the drug rapidly from the body and good nursing care.

Reference

Morrow JI, Routledge PA. Poisoning with anticonvulsants. *Adv Drug React Acute Poisoning Rev* 1989; **8**: 97–109.

Phenothiazines and related neuroleptic agents

Aliphatic phenothiazines
Chlorpromazine
Promazine

Piperazine phenothiazines
Fluphenazine
Perphenazine
Prochlorperazine
Trifluoperazine

Piperidine phenothiazines
Mesoridazine
Thioridazine

Thioxanthines
Chlorprothixene
Flupenthixol

Butyrophenones
Haloperidol
Droperidol

General considerations

Phenothiazines, thioxanthenes and butyrophenones have common pharmacological actions although the third group is chemically unrelated to the other two. Despite their widespread use for treatment of psychiatric illness, acute overdosage with these compounds is relatively uncommon. Chlorpromazine, thioridazine, trifluoperazine and prochlorperazine are most frequently encountered. Occasionally self-poisoning with a combined preparation containing perphenazine and a tricyclic antidepressant is encountered and the toxicity of the antidepressant dominates, although some features may be potentiated by the phenothiazine (e.g. cardiotoxicity).

Phenothiazines are perhaps more important in the context of self-poisoning because of the disabling parkinsonian features which long-term use has caused in some schizophrenic patients. They are commonly being treated with injections of fluphenazine or flupenthixol with or without oral phenothiazines. While the drugs may be controlling florid psychotic illness, their adverse effects are occasionally so severe that they may be contributing to the difficulty the patient has in coping with life, whether or not anticholinergic drugs such as orphenadrine and benztropine are also given.

Features

Overdosage with phenothiazines and related drugs causes CNS depression but profound coma and respiratory failure are uncommon. On the other hand they produce disproportionately severe hypotension and hypothermia. Some conscious patients show acute dystonic reactions including oculogyric crises, torticollis and orolingual dyskinesias, particularly with trifluoperazine, prochlorperazine and haloperidol. Other parkinsonian features are usually the result of long-term therapy rather than acute overdosage. Convulsions may occur. Acute renal failure secondary to interstitial nephritis has been reported after overdosage with chlorprothixene.

A tachycardia is often present but conduction abnormalities and dysrhythmias are rare, although well-documented, particularly with thioridazine and mesoridazine. They may resemble those seen with tricyclic antidepressants. The PR, QRS and QT intervals may be prolonged and, rarely, bifid T waves are present. The most common reported dysrhythmias are ventricular tachycardia and fibrillation. Rarely, haloperidol will cause similar cardiotoxicity. Acute pulmonary oedema has been reported.

Death is usually due to cardiac effects.

Management

It is doubtful if there is merit in attempting to empty the stomach. Repeated doses of oral activated charcoal should be given. Treatment thereafter is symptomatic. Hypotension usually responds to supportive measures and intravascular volume expansion is seldom necessary. Cardiac dysrhythmias due to phenothiazines pose difficult therapeutic problems. Limited experience suggests that digoxin, phenytoin and lignocaine are of no value but these and other antidysrhythmic drugs may have to be tried in life-threatening situations. Attention should first be paid to correcting hypoxia, acid–base disturbances and the plasma potassium concentration.

Dystonic reactions can be abolished rapidly by intramuscular injection of benztropine (1–2 mg for an adult), procyclidine (5–10 mg for an adult) or diphenhydramine (2 mg/kg body weight to a maximum of 50 mg) for a child.

Forced diuresis, haemodialysis and haemoperfusion are of no value.

References

Henderson RA, Lane S, Henry JA. Life-threatening ventricular arrhythmia (torsades de pointes) after haloperidol overdose. *Hum Exp Toxicol* 1991; **10**: 59–62.

Li C, Gefter WB. Acute pulmonary edema induced by overdosage of phenothiazines. *Chest* 1992; **101**: 102–104.

Marrs-Simon PA, Zell-Kanter M, Kendzierski DL *et al*. Cardiotoxic manifestations of mesoridazine overdose. *Ann Emerg Med* 1988; **17**: 1074–1078.

Reid W, Harrower ADB. Cardiac arrest after apparent recovery from an overdose of chlorpromazine. *Br Med J* 1984; **288**: 1880.

Scheithauer W, Ulrich W, Kovarik *et al*. Acute oliguria associated with chlorprothixine overdosage. *Nephron* 1988; **48**: 71–73.

Phenoxyacetate and related herbicides

2,4-dichlorophenoxyacetic acid (2,4-D)
4-(2,4-dichlorophenoxy)butyric acid (2,4-DB)
2-(2,4-dichlorophenoxy)propionic acid (2,4-DP, DCPP, dichlorprop)
2,4,5-trichlorophenoxyacetic acid (2,4,5-T)
2-(2,4,5-trichlorophenoxy)propionic acid (2,4,5-TP, fenoprop)
4-chloro-2-methylphenoxyacetic acid (MCPA)
4-(4-chloro-2-methylphenoxy)butyric acid (MCPB)
2-(4-chloro-2-methylphenoxy)propionic acid (MCPP, mecoprop)

General considerations

Phenoxyacetate herbicides are used widely in agriculture for the control of broad-leaved weeds growing among cereals and are also available to the public for use in gardens. Though systemic effects can follow absorption through the bronchial tree, most instances of serious poisoning have been due to deliberate ingestion. Few cases have been reported. These herbicides are often coformulated with dicamba which has low toxicity and ioxynil and bromoxynil which uncouple oxidative phosphorylation.

Features

Initially there is burning in the mouth and throat followed by nausea, vomiting and abdominal pain. The face may be flushed and there is often profuse sweating and fever. The most impressive effects are CNS depression with drowsiness leading to deep, prolonged coma. Hyperventilation, carpopedal spasm, hypotension, hypoglycaemia, metabolic acidosis and pulmonary oedema may develop. Increased muscle tone and hyperreflexia may be present initially. The plasma urea may be elevated despite a good urinary output and muscle damage is reflected in raised serum activities of lactic dehydrogenase, creatine phosphokinase, aldolase and aspartate and alanine aminotransferases. Electromyographic changes consistent with a mild proximal myopathy were found in 1 survivor 6 days after ingestion. Electrocardiogram abnormalities have been reported.

Management

The stomach should be emptied and any necessary supportive measures instituted. The phenoxyacetate herbicides are moderately strong acids and alkalinization of the urine by intravenous infusion of sodium bicarbonate (see salicylate poisoning, p. 208) considerably enhances elimination of 2,4-D and dichlorprop and, to a lesser extent, mecoprop. It should therefore be started as soon as possible if the patient is unconscious or is acidaemic. The effect of alkaline diuresis on excretion of other compounds in this group may be less and the elimination of ioxynil is not changed. There are no published data on the efficacy of haemodialysis, though one would expect these compounds to be freely dialysable.

References

Flanagan RJ, Meredith TJ, Ruprah M *et al.* Alkaline diuresis for acute poisoning with chlorophenoxy herbicides and ioxynil. *Lancet* 1990; **335**: 454–458.
Kancir CB, Andersen C, Olesen AS. Marked hypocalcemia in a fatal poisoning with chlorinated phenoxy acid derivatives. *Clin Toxicol* 1988; **26**: 257–264.

Phenytoin

General considerations

Phenytoin (diphenylhydantoin) is widely used as an anticonvulsant and is commonly taken in deliberate overdosage by epileptics and their relatives and close friends.

Features

The features of phenytoin poisoning include nausea, vomiting, nystagmus, dysarthria, ataxia, drowsiness and, rarely, coma. Temporary abolition of the ocular responses to head rotation (the doll's-head reflex) and ice-water stimulation of the ears at a time when the patients were able to carry out commands has been reported. The mechanism of this phenomenon is not understood. Paradoxically, convulsions may be a complication.

Plasma phenytoin concentrations

Plasma phenytoin concentrations can be measured readily and values of up to 112 mg/l (445 µmol/l) have been reported after acute overdosage. About 90% of plasma phenytoin is protein-bound and at high concentrations the half-life is very long because of saturation of the drug-metabolizing enzymes. There is no merit in measuring plasma phenytoin concentrations as an emergency but daily measurement can be of value in estimating the duration of toxicity and timing the reintroduction of regular therapy in epileptics (the therapeutic range is 8–15 mg/l or 32–60 µmol/l).

Management

There is no specific treatment for phenytoin intoxication. Repeated doses of oral activated charcoal should be given to shorten the plasma half-life of the drug and supportive measures may be necessary if the patient is unconscious. Intravenous fluids should be given if nausea and vomiting are severe. Attempts to force a diuresis will not increase phenytoin excretion. Similarly, peritoneal dialysis and haemodialysis are of no value. In epileptics, plasma phenytoin concentrations should be monitored to ensure that they do not fall so rapidly and to such an extent that convulsions occur.

Prognosis

The vast majority of patients poisoned with phenytoin survive although the plasma half-life of the drug is such that recovery may take several days. Occasional deaths have been reported and some investigators believe that permanent neurological damage can occur after a single acute exposure.

References

Larsen JR, Larsen LS. Clinical features and management of poisoning due to phenytoin. *Med Toxicol Adv Drug Exp* 1989; **4**: 229–245.

Masur H, Fahrendorf G, Oberwittler C *et al.* Cerebellar atrophy following acute intoxication with phenytoin. *Neurology* 1990; **40**: 1800.

Murphy JM, Motiwala R, Devinski O. Phenytoin intoxication. *South Med J* 1991; **84**: 1199–1204.

Potassium chloride

General considerations

Acute overdosage with potassium chloride is surprisingly uncommon considering the vast quantities prescribed. However, deaths have been reported in children and adults after accidental and deliberate ingestion of large numbers of tablets, including 'slow-release' formulations. Dangerous hyperkalaemia has also followed the ingestion of salt substitutes. The principal toxic effect of potassium is on the myocardium and depends on the concentration gradient across the cell membrane and the rate at which it changes rather than the absolute plasma concentration. Thus patients who develop hyperkalaemia slowly are at less risk than those who attain similar levels acutely.

Features

Initially the patient may appear deceptively unaffected by an acute overdose of potassium chloride. Nausea and vomiting are common within a short time of ingestion but give no indication of the severity of poisoning. The most helpful investigations are the plasma potassium concentration and the electrocardiogram. The electrocardiogram manifestations of hyperkalaemia comprise peaking of the T waves, reduction of the amplitude of the P wave and PR prolongation till the P wave is lost in the preceding T. The QRS complex widens progressively and in severe poisoning may resemble a sine wave. Ventricular tachycardia may occur but death is usually due to asystole.

Management

The plasma potassium and urea must be measured urgently immediately on admission and at frequent intervals thereafter, taking care not to haemolyse the samples. Arterial blood gas analysis should also be carried out to detect any metabolic acidosis.

The electrocardiogram must be monitored continuously. Evidence of cardiac toxicity requires immediate action and should take precedence over measures to prevent further absorption of potassium. Calcium gluconate (10–20 ml of a 10% solution for an adult) should be given intravenously to stabilize the myocardial cell membrane while the plasma potassium is being reduced and is indicated if there is QRS widening.

The potassium gradient across the cell membrane is reduced by shifting potassium from the extracellular fluid into the cell by giving dextrose (100 ml of a 50% solution) intravenously. Soluble insulin (10–20 units) by the same route has been recommended but should not be necessary, except perhaps in diabetics, since the glucose ought to stimulate endogenous insulin release. Intravenous sodium bicarbonate (50 mmol or more) should be given to correct any metabolic acidosis and to produce an alkalaemia, thereby facilitating the movement of potassium into cells. The extracellular potassium concentration can also be reduced by increasing elimination of potassium. The simplest way to do this is to induce a diuresis by giving intravenous fluids and frusemide if the patient's cardiac state and renal function permit. If this is not possible urgent haemodialysis (or, if that is not immediately available, peritoneal dialysis) should be considered.

Once the patient's cardiac state has been stabilized the stomach should be emptied and an ion exchange resin such as calcium or sodium polystyrene sulphonate left in the stomach. The latter may also be given rectally.

Slow-release potassium preparations release potassium over 3–6 hours or even longer and in severe poisoning the use of whole-bowel irrigation (p. 42) to eliminate tablets beyond reach of the stomach tube should be considered.

References

Saxena K. Clinical features and management of poisoning due to potassium chloride. *Med Toxicol Adv Drug Exp* 1989; **4**: 429–443.
Steedman DJ. Poisoning with sustained release potassium. *Arch Emerg Med* 1988; **5**: 206–211.

Primidone

General considerations

Primidone is an anticonvulsant which is toxic in its own right, apart from any contribution from its two active metabolites, phenobarbitone and phenylethylmalonamide. Acute primidone overdosage is uncommon.

Features

The features of primidone poisoning are those of CNS depression. Drowsiness, dysarthria, ataxia and coarse nystagmus are common and the patient may behave in a disinhibited manner. Rarely, coma, hypotonia, hyporeflexia, hypothermia, hypotension and respiratory depression may occur. A distinctive feature is the presence of whorls of shimmering white crystals in the urine. Surprisingly, renal failure has not been described.

Plasma primidone concentrations

Plasma primidone concentrations up to 100 mg/l have been reported after acute overdosage and decline with a half-life of about 15 hours. As the primidone concentration falls the plasma concentrations of phenobarbitone and phenylethylmalonamide frequently rise although the patient may be improving clinically.

Management

There is no specific treatment for primidone poisoning. Repeated doses of oral activated charcoal should be given to shorten the plasma half-life of the drug. Supportive measures should be implemented if necessary.

References

Lehmann DF. Primidone crystalluria following overdose. *Med Toxicol* 1987; **2**: 383–387.

Morrow JI, Routledge PA. Poisoning with anticonvulsants. *Adv Drug React Acute Poisoning Rev* 1989; **8**: 97–109.

Quinine

General considerations

Quinine sulphate is widely prescribed for the prevention of nocturnal cramp and accidental and deliberate acute overdosage still occurs from time to time. Few cases are now due to attempts to induce abortion. Quinine is an alkaloid obtained from the bark of the cinchona tree which grows in some regions of South America. Cinchonism is the collective term for the symptoms of quinine intoxication.

Features

The early features of quinine poisoning are nausea, vomiting, tinnitus and deafness. The skin is usually flushed, warm and moist.

Visual impairment is the most common dramatic feature and includes all degrees of severity from blurring to complete blindness developing over a few hours. The mechanism involved is not clear but there is increasing support for a direct effect on the retina rather than ischaemia secondary to quinine-induced arteriolar constriction. The pupils dilate and become progressively less reactive to light as visual acuity decreases. The fundi are usually normal for the first day or two but by the third or fourth day after ingestion there is often retinal oedema, peripapillary oedema and attenuation of the retinal arterioles. Perimetry usually demonstrates severe constriction of the visual fields.

Coma, convulsions, respiratory failure, hypotension, cardiac dys-rhythmias and disseminated intravascular coagulation have been reported after ingestion of very large quantities.

Plasma quinine concentrations

Serum or plasma quinine concentrations of up to 25 mg/l have been reported after acute poisoning and those above 15 mg/l at some time carry an increased risk of ocular and cardiac toxicity.

Management

The stomach should be emptied if the overdose has been taken within the preceding 4 hours. Repeated doses of oral activated charcoal should be started as soon as possible since there is some evidence that they shorten the plasma half-life of the toxin which is otherwise about 26 hours after overdosage. Less than 5% of quinine is excreted unchanged in the urine and it has a large volume of distribution; forced acid diuresis, haemodialysis, charcoal haemoperfusion and exchange transfusion have been shown to be ineffective. Rare cases with coma, convulsions and cardiac dysrhythmias will require appropriate supportive care.

Various measures have been used in attempts to improve impaired visual acuity but the available evidence suggests that none, including stellate ganglion block, is effective. Repeat-dose charcoal to reduce plasma quinine concentrations as rapidly as possible is the measure most likely to minimize ocular toxicity.

Prognosis

Death from quinine poisoning is rare and only likely to occur in patients with severe CNS or cardiac toxicity. Visual impairment is the only serious long-term complication and though improvement tends to occur, even without treatment, some constriction of the peripheral fields with tunnel vision is likely to persist. Optic atrophy develops in these cases.

References

Dyson EH, Proudfoot AT, Bateman DN. Quinine amblyopia: is current management appropriate? *Clin Toxicol* 1985–86; **23**: 571–578.

Schonwald S, Shannon M. Unsuspected quinine intoxication presenting as acute deafness and mutism. *Am J Emerg Med* 1991; **9**: 318–320.

Salicylates

General considerations

The prevalence of both accidental and deliberate self-poisoning with salicylates has declined sharply in the last decade or so as paracetamol (acetaminophen) has become the standard domestic analgesic. The mechanisms of many of the manifestations of salicylate toxicity remain incompletely understood and it still presents diagnostic and therapeutic challenges. More than 150, 250 and 500 mg/kg body weight is likely to produce mild, moderate and severe poisoning respectively. Fortunately methyl salicylate (oil of wintergreen) poisoning is now seldom encountered since it is several times more toxic than similar amounts of other salicylates.

Diagnosis of salicylate poisoning is usually straightforward but recent reports have drawn attention to difficulties when it complicates treatment of febrile illnesses in childhood. To some extent therapeutic intoxication results from the dose-dependent pharmacokinetics of salicylic acid. Salicylates are well-absorbed and aspirin (acetylsalicylic acid) is rapidly hydrolysed to salicylic acid which is metabolized comparatively slowly to salicyluric acid and salicyl, acyl and phenolic glucuronides. The enzymes responsible are readily saturated within the range of therapeutic doses. Accumulation of salicylic acid is therefore very likely with large doses or frequent repetition of doses. The risk of therapeutic poisoning is increased if the hyperventilation, sweating, flushing and fever are erroneously attributed to the underlying illness and interpreted as an indication for further salicylate.

Salicylate poisoning may also occur by percutaneous absorption when salicylic acid ointment is applied extensively as a keratolytic agent.

Features

The clinical features of salicylate intoxication vary with age, young children tending to tolerate overdosage less well than older children and adults.

Mild and moderate poisoning
Salicylates commonly cause tinnitus, deafness, nausea and vomiting. Hyperventilation results from stimulation of the respiratory centre. Cardiac output is also increased with peripheral vasodilatation, bounding pulses and profuse sweating. Hyperpyrexia occurs in children but is seldom seen in adults. Some degree of dehydration is common.

Hypoglycaemia occasionally complicates salicylate poisoning in children but is very rare in adults. Significant prolongation of the prothrombin time does not occur. Other unusual complications include gastric haemorrhage and tetany.

Young women in particular may develop subconjunctival haemorrhage and petechiae, usually on the eyelids, but occasionally more extensively over the face and neck. The precise cause of these is uncertain but they are probably due to a combination of reduced platelet stickiness and raised venous pressure associated with retching, vomiting and struggling during gastric lavage. They do not indicate a serious blood dyscrasia. Investigation is unnecessary and patient and relatives should merely be assured that the spots will fade in a few days. Despite the frequent occurrence of subconjunctival or dermal haemorrhage, retinal haemorrhages have not been reported.

Severe poisoning
Severe poisoning is distinguished by the presence of CNS features including delirium, extreme agitation, confusion, coma and convulsions.

Impairment of consciousness is most commonly encountered in children below the age of 2 years and is rare in older children and adults. Indeed it is failure to lose consciousness together with the misery of salicylism which ultimately drives some adults to seek treatment late after overdosage. CNS features in adult salicylate poisoning indicate a grave prognosis.

Acidaemia and non-cardiogenic pulmonary oedema are common in severe intoxication (see acid–base abnormalities). Rarely, there may be cerebral oedema and oliguria and renal failure despite an adequate circulating blood volume. The latter suggests that there may be inappropriate secretion of antidiuretic hormone.

Acid–base abnormalities

Complex acid–base disturbances complicate salicylate intoxication and the resultant arterial hydrogen ion concentration is vital in determining the distribution of the drug. Since salicylates are weak acids, alkalaemia (reduced arterial hydrogen ion concentration or high pH) tends to keep the drug within the vascular compartment while acidaemia (raised hydrogen ion concentration or low pH) facilitates movement into the tissues, particularly the brain. Patients with CNS features are therefore usually acidaemic, although with very high plasma salicylate concentrations it is possible to develop the same features despite being alkalaemic. Reduction of the venous bicarbonate may indicate a metabolic acidosis but is more commonly the consequence of a respiratory alkalosis. Accurate assessment of the acid–base disturbance demands arterial blood gas analysis.

The arterial hydrogen ion concentration in salicylate poisoning depends on the balance of two opposing effects. Respiratory stimulation causes hyperventilation, reduction in $Pa\text{CO}_2$ and a respiratory alkalosis; uncoupling of oxidative phosphorylation results in production of lactate and other organic acids of intermediary metabolism and a metabolic acidosis. However, the traditional view that salicylate-induced uncoupling of oxidative phosphorylation is responsible for increased oxygen uptake, carbon dioxide production and basal metabolic rate has recently been challenged. Whatever the truth, children under the age of 4 years have a dominant metabolic component and often become acidaemic. In older children and adults the respiratory effect usually dominates and arterial hydrogen ion concentration remains normal or is reduced. In a small proportion of adults however acidaemia results and, as in young children, is commonly associated with impairment of consciousness.

It is traditionally held that the acid–base changes of salicylate poisoning occur in sequence, an initial respiratory alkalosis being followed by a metabolic acidosis. However in some cases acidaemia develops within 3 hours of acute poisoning and the respiratory alkalosis must be very brief or absent. The acid–base changes are not related to the magnitude of the plasma salicylate concentration.

Plasma salicylate concentrations

Plasma salicylate concentrations can be measured simply and rapidly. The features of salicylism are present at concentrations of 300 mg/l (2.2 mmol/l) or more. Plasma concentrations exceed 700 mg/l (5.1 mmol/l) in about 4% of overdose cases. Rarely values as high as 1700 mg/l (12.3 mmol/l) are obtained.

Plasma salicylate concentrations increase after admission in about 10% of cases probably due to absorption of drug flushed from the stomach into the small bowel during gastric lavage. It may therefore be necessary to measure the plasma salicylate concentration again a few hours after the initial estimation.

As indicated above, coma in adult salicylate overdosage is far from common and the indiscriminate measurement of plasma salicylate concentrations in all unconscious poisoned patients cannot be justified.

Management

General

The stomach should be emptied if more than 4.5 g has been taken by an adult or 2 g by a child within 4 hours and oral activated charcoal given. The plasma salicylate concentration should be measured in patients with symptoms. Arterial blood gas analysis is indicated in clinically severe poisoning and in those with high plasma salicylate concentrations. It is unnecessary to prescribe vitamin K routinely.

Increasing elimination of absorbed salicylate

Minor toxicity. Children and adults with concentrations of less than 350 mg/l (2.5 mmol/l) and 450 mg/l (3.3 mmol/l) respectively do not usually require more than an increase in oral fluid intake.

Moderate toxicity. The technique which permits optimum elimination compatible with safety in children with plasma salicylate concentrations above 350 mg/l (2.5 mmol/l) and adults above 450 mg/l (3.3 mmol/l) but below 700 mg/l (5.1 mmol/l) is controversial. Repeated doses of oral activated charcoal should be given since they significantly shorten the plasma half-life of salicylate in those in whom metabolism is fully saturated. However, it is not clear whether repeated oral charcoal is sufficient on its own and it is probably advisable to combine it with measures to alkalinize the urine. The latter usually requires intravenous sodium bicarbonate and 0.5 l of a 1.26% solution hourly for 3 hours should be sufficient for adults. Acetazolamide has also been given to induce an alkaline urine but while it is undoubtedly effective and works rapidly, it cannot be recommended since it also produces a systemic acidosis which could enhance the toxicity of salicylate.

Severe poisoning, as defined in clinical terms (see above), or by the presence of acidaemia or plasma salicylate concentrations exceeding 700 mg/l (5.1 mmol/l) carries a mortality of about 5% and should prompt consideration of urgent referral for haemodialysis. Haemoperfusion effectively removes salicylate but is illogical since it does not aid management of the metabolic abnormalities. Patients who do not show features of neurotoxicity but who are acidaemic or have high levels may be closely monitored clinically and biochemically. Some of them will recover without dialysis but others deteriorate rapidly and are best observed in centres with appropriate facilities. In these cases, acidaemia should be corrected as a matter of urgency and repeated oral charcoal given. Forced diuresis is likely to precipitate fatal pulmonary oedema and is contraindicated.

Supportive measures
In life-threatening poisoning, curarization and passive hyperventilation may have a temporary role while initiating appropriate measures to enhance the elimination of the drug. Hyperventilation, often gross, is invariably present and the work of breathing may be an important contributor to lactic acidosis and acidaemia. It is also worth giving glucose (25 g intravenously) since animal studies have shown that brain glucose concentrations may be severely reduced despite normal plasma levels.

References

Chapman BJ, Proudfoot AT. Adult salicylate poisoning: deaths and outcome in patients with high plasma salicylate concentrations. *Q J Med* 1989; **72**: 699–707.
Proudfoot AT. Salicylates and salicylamide. In *Poisoning and Drug Overdose*, 2nd edn (Haddad LM, Winchester JF, eds). WB Saunders, 1990, pp 909–920.

Scombrotoxic fish poisoning

General considerations

Scombrotoxic fish poisoning is due to the accumulation of a heat-stable toxin in the flesh of red meat fish such as tuna, mackerel, bonito, skipjack and dolphin (mahimahi) which has been stored at insufficiently low temperatures. The spoiled fish usually contains excessively high concentrations of histamine which accumulate due to the action of bacterial decarboxylase on histidine. A variety of bacteria including species of *Proteus, Escherichia coli* and *Salmonella* have been incriminated. However scombrotoxic poisoning may occur in the absence of high fish histamine content and conversely when histamine concentrations are high, poisoning does not necessarily develop.

Similar poisoning has occurred after ingestion of scombroid fish by patients taking isoniazid which inhibits histaminase.

Features

Symptoms usually start within 3 hours and often within a few minutes. Most can be explained by the action of histamine on smooth muscle and include flushing, particularly over the face, trunk and arms, stuffy nose, burning of the mouth, throbbing headache, palpitations, pruritus, nausea, abdominal pain and diarrhoea. In severe cases breathlessness and wheeze may occur. Urticaria is uncommon.

Treatment

Treatment is seldom necessary and recovery is usually complete in 12 hours. Symptomatic treatment may be indicated in rare severe cases.

References

Easthaugh J, Shepherd S. Infectious and toxic syndromes from fish and shellfish consumption. *Arch Intern Med* 1989; **149**: 1735–1740.
Taylor SL, Stratton JE, Nordlee JA. Histamine poisoning (scombroid fish poisoning): an allergy-like intoxication. *Clin Toxicol* 1989; **27**: 225–240.

Shellfish poisoning

General considerations

Paralytic or neurotoxic shellfish poisoning is uncommon. Sporadic cases and minor outbreaks have been reported from various parts of the world including Alaska, Canada, Western Europe and the UK. Poisoning usually follows ingestion of mussels and occasionally cockles or clams and is due to a water-soluble, heat-stable toxin known as saxitoxin. It is most likely to occur in spring and summer when a sudden increase in sea temperature leads to rapid multiplication of dino-flagellates, particularly *Gonyaulax tamarensis*, which discolour surface water leading to the description of waterbloom or red tides. These organisms are filtered by the molluscs which thereby concentrate the toxin.

Features

Symptoms may start within as short a period as 20 min or as long as 10 hours but generally within 3 or 4 hours. Circumoral paraesthesiae and numbness are very common and may also occur in the fingers and toes and spread up the limbs. Frequently there is a feeling of dizziness, ataxia or floating and generalized muscle weakness may give rise to difficulty in moving and breathing. Vomiting and headache are less frequent features.

Management

There is no specific treatment for paralytic shellfish poisoning. Supportive measures are all that is required. The most important point is to ensure adequate respiration. Assisted ventilation may be required in severe cases. Complete recovery may be expected if the patient survives 24 hours.

Reference

Easthaugh J, Shepherd S. Infectious and toxic syndromes from fish and shellfish consumption. *Arch Intern Med* 1989; **149**: 1735–1740.

Smoke

General considerations

People who are involved in fires are at serious risk even if they escape skin burns and thermal injury to the upper respiratory tract. Asphyxia is a hazard if the fire uses the available oxygen. Smoke is another potentially lethal cause of injury since it contains particles and toxic gases which, unlike heat, readily reach the alveoli. The gases present at fires vary considerably according to the materials involved and the temperature of combustion. Hydrogen chloride (from polyvinyl wall, floor and furnishing coverings), isocyanates (from polyurethane foams), phosgene, acrolein and a variety of aldehydes may cause alveolar damage and impair gas exchange while carbon monoxide reduces the oxygen-carrying capacity of the blood without causing chemical pulmonary damage and hydrogen cyanide prevents cellular oxygen utilization. The role of inhaled particles (mainly soot) in the pathogenesis of pulmonary lesions has not yet been elucidated but may be unimportant.

Many patients will have preexisting chronic obstructive airways disease from cigarette smoking. Many fires arise through smoking in bed, occasionally while under the influence of alcohol or drugs.

Features

Most patients who present to physicians will have minimal or no burns. Those with even minimal facial burns, singeing of the hair, eyebrows and eyelashes must be observed very carefully since they are at risk of thermal injury to the upper respiratory tract and may develop delayed severe respiratory obstruction due either to laryngeal oedema or expectoration of large sheets of desquamated mucosa. Damage does not occur beyond the main bronchi because air temperature drops very rapidly after inhalation.

Many patients will be covered in soot and smell strongly of smoke. Depending on the acridity of the smoke the eyes may sting and stream and there may be a metallic taste in the mouth. The voice may be hoarse and the throat sore and inflamed. Cough, wheeze, breathlessness and chest tightness are common complaints. The sputum often contains large amounts of soot. Rhonchi and crepitations may be heard on auscultation. Central cyanosis may be obvious. Many patients will have significant concentrations of carboxyhaemoglobin in their blood without the skin showing the 'typical' cherry red colour.

Arterial blood gas analysis immediately on arrival at hospital often reveals much more marked hypoxia than would be suspected from the symptoms and signs, unless oxygen has been given en route from the fire. Pa_{CO_2} is usually slightly reduced, reflecting hyperventilation, and the hydrogen ion concentration may be reduced or increased depending on whether hypoxia has been of sufficient severity and duration to produce a metabolic acidosis.

Carboxyhaemoglobin concentrations between 10 and 50% are common but higher values are usually found only in fatal cases. The concentration on arrival at hospital may underestimate the severity of exposure since carboxyhaemoglobin will tend to dissociate as soon as exposure to carbon monoxide ceases, especially if oxygen is given. Plasma concentrations of cyanide and other toxins absorbed by inhalation during fires have been measured but are seldom sufficiently high on their own to cause death. They probably potentiate other factors to increase morbidity and mortality.

The majority of smoke inhalation victims have normal chest X-rays but some show bronchial wall thickening, subglottic oedema, or have focal pulmonary infiltrates which clear in about 3 days, diffuse patchy opacities (which tend to resolve more slowly) or changes in keeping with pulmonary oedema. The radiographic appearances correlate poorly with the degree of hypoxia and carboxyhaemoglobin concentrations which are better guides to the severity of smoke inhalation.

The electrocardiogram may show tachycardia and ischaemic changes.

Management

Reversal of toxic effects starts the moment the victim is removed from the smoke. Lives may be saved at the scene of the fire by simple measures to establish a clear airway and assist ventilation before transfer to hospital. High concentrations of oxygen in the inspired air should be given at high flow rates in the ambulance. These measures should be continued till the adequacy of ventilation and severity of exposure have been assessed by arterial blood gas analysis, measurement of the carboxyhaemoglobin level and the findings on chest X-ray. Seek the advice of an anaesthetist if there is the slightest doubt about the presence of thermal injury to the upper respiratory tract; laryngoscopy or fibreoptic bronchoscopy may be required to determine the full extent of the damage and appropriate respiratory management. Carbon monoxide poisoning should be managed as described on p. 89.

Greatest doubt centres on the presence of concomitant cyanide poisoning. Unfortunately, significant involvement of cyanide in smoke inhalation can only be surmised; there is no qualitative or quantitative laboratory test to aid the clinician. However, the concentrations usually found are seldom toxic and cyanide should only be a matter for concern in patients with the most severe consequences of smoke inhalation; stable patients should not be treated with cyanide antidotes which are inherently toxic and may make matters worse rather than better.

References

Baud FJ, Barriot P, Toffis V et al. Elevated blood cyanide concentrations in victims of smoke inhalation. N Engl J Med 1991; 325: 1761–1766.

Beritic T. The challenge of fire effluents. Br Med J 1990; 300: 696–698.

Langford RM, Armstrong RF. Algorithm for managing injury from smoke inhalation. Br Med J 1989; 299: 902–904.

Lee MJ, O'Connell DJ. The plain chest radiograph after acute smoke inhalation. Clin Radiol 1988; 39: 39–37.

Peitzman AB, Shires GT, Teixdor HS et al. Smoke inhalation injury: evaluation of radiographic manifestations and pulmonary dysfunction. J Trauma 1989; 29: 1232–1239.

Prien T, Trabor DL. Toxic smoke compounds and inhalation injury. Burns 1988; 14: 451–460.

Soaps, household detergents and fabric conditioners

General considerations

Soaps, household detergents and fabric conditioners are commonly ingested by toddlers. Soaps comprise sodium and potassium salts of fatty acids obtained from edible fats. Synthetic detergents are complex formulations of a variety of chemicals including surface acting agents (usually anionic or non-ionic varieties), mild alkalis (sodium silicate or sodium triphosphate) which comprise the bulk of washing powders, and bleaches (sodium hypochlorite or sodium perborate) in addition to perfumes, proteolytic enzymes, whiteners, stabilizers etc. The relative amounts vary according to the nature of the material to be cleaned and the conditions under which it is to be used (e.g. temperature, degree of mechanical agitation, etc.). The principal ingredient of fabric conditioners (intended to make clothes soft and fluffy) is a cationic detergent, often di-alkyl, di-methyl ammonium chloride. Fortunately the complexities of detergent formulations are clinically relatively unimportant.

Cationic detergents such as benzalkonium chloride are potentially very toxic.

Features

Only a minority of children who ingest these products develop symptoms. Except in rare cases where aspiration into the lungs occurs, features of ingestion are confined to the alimentary tract. Nausea, vomiting and diarrhoea are common but abdominal pain, haematemesis or rectal bleeding seldom occur. There may be discomfort or pain in the mouth but ulceration of the mucosa is unusual, even when the most alkaline of these products (granular and liquid automatic dishwashing detergents) are swallowed.

Solutions containing 10% or more of benzalkonium chloride are likely to cause corrosive lesions of the upper alimentary tract. Features of systemic toxicity include coma, convulsions, muscle weakness, respiratory failure, metabolic acidosis and renal failure.

Management

There is no specific treatment for ingestion of soaps and detergents. It is unnecessary to empty the stomach. A good fluid intake should be ensured and demulcents such as milk may be helpful. It is seldom necessary to refer children to hospital after ingestion of these products.

Local lesions due to cationic detergent toxicity should be treated as other corrosive lesions (p. 108) and systemic toxicity supportively.

Prognosis

Symptoms almost always disappear well within 24 hours.

References

Krenzelok EP. Liquid automatic dishwashing detergents: a profile of toxicity. *Ann Emerg Med* 1989; **18**: 60–63.

van Berkel M, de Wolff FA. Survival after acute benzalkonium chloride poisoning. *Hum Toxicol* 1988; **7**: 191–193,

Theophylline and sympathomimetic bronchodilators

Theophylline and its derivatives
Aminophylline
Choline theophyllinate
Theophylline

Selective beta$_2$-adrenoceptor stimulants
Salbutamol
Terbutaline

Others
Ephedrine
Orciprenaline
Pseudoephedrine

General considerations

Deliberate self-poisoning with bronchodilators probably occurs more often than the literature would suggest and therapeutic overdosage is also common. In addition, some patients with respiratory diseases become dependent on the CNS stimulant effects of bronchodilators and take them orally or by inhalation to gross excess. Despite the increasing number of newer drugs, those listed above remain the ones most commonly encountered in overdosage.

Theophylline is by far the most toxic of the bronchodilators. Some older, but still popular, bronchodilator formulations combine ephedrine (an alpha- and beta-adrenergic agonist which occurs naturally in a wide variety of plants) with a xanthine derivative (theophylline or aminophylline) which potentiate each other when taken in overdosage.

Features

It is particularly important to appreciate that most oral theophylline preparations currently marketed are of the sustained-release variety. Serious toxicity may therefore not be apparent until 12–24 hours after ingestion.

Gastrointestinal
Theophylline derivatives cause marked gastrointestinal irritation with nausea, intractable vomiting and occasionally diarrhoea. Haematemesis is also common and may be severe. Ephedrine, salbutamol and terbutaline are much less likely to produce these effects.

Neuromuscular
All the bronchodilators considered here cause CNS stimulation. The patient becomes restless, anxious, hyperactive and talks rapidly. Dilatation of the pupils is common and tremor and hyperventilation are integral parts of the increase in arousal. Myoclonus, erratic jerky movements of the limbs, increased muscle tone and exaggerated reflexes usually precede convulsions which may be generalized or focal. The generalized increase in muscular activity commonly causes rhabdomyolysis and hyperpyrexia. Impairment of consciousness may eventually occur.

Cardiovascular
A tachycardia is invariable, even in mild poisoning. The blood pressure may be slightly raised in the initial phase but falls later. Supraventricular and ventricular ectopic beats presage more serious tachydysrhythmias, including ventricular fibrillation. It is uncertain to what extent the cardiac effects are due to the drugs themselves or to the increased endogenous catecholamine secretion they cause.

Metabolic
A number of complex, inter-related metabolic disturbances accompany overdosage with xanthines and ephedrine. In the initial phases hyperventilation leads to a respiratory alkalosis but a metabolic acidosis develops as poisoning becomes more severe. Hyperglycaemia and glycosuria result from increased secretion of catecholamines which, together with theophylline, also stimulate lipolysis with subsequent elevation of plasma free fatty acid concentrations. Production of cyclic adenosine monophosphate is stimulated by ephedrine and its breakdown reduced by theophylline which is a phosphodiesterase inhibitor. These drugs therefore potentiate the effects of endogenous catecholamines causing hyperinsulinaemia and severe hypokalaemia as potassium is driven into cells.

Assessment of the severity of poisoning

The following system has been proposed for grading the severity of theophylline intoxication but has not been applied to poisoning with other bronchodilators:

Severity grade	Features
1	Vomiting, abdominal pain, diarrhoea, nervousness, tremor, sinus tachycardia >120 beats/min, plasma potassium <3.5 mmol/l but >2.5 mmol/l.
2	Haematemesis, lethargy or disorientation, supraventricular dysrhythmias, frequent ventricular ectopics, mean blood pressure 60 mmHg but responsive to standard therapy, plasma potassium <2.5 mmol/l, arterial hydrogen ion concentration >63 nmol/l (pH <7.20) or <25 nmol/l (pH >7.60), rhabdomyolysis.
3	Seizure (non-repetitive), sustained ventricular tachycardia, mean blood pressure <60 mmHg and unresponsive to standard therapy.
4	Status epilepticus, ventricular fibrillation, cardiac arrest.

Plasma concentrations of theophylline

Plasma concentrations of theophylline can be measured by high performance liquid chromatography and with therapeutic doses are usually of the order of 10–20 mg/l (77–154 µmol/l). Theophylline concentrations seldom exceed 300 mg/l (2300 µmol/l) after acute overdosage and, with sustained-release formulations, peak concentrations are only attained after 8–12 hours. The plasma half-life of theophylline in such cases is about 9 hours.

Management

Patients with theophylline overdosage require particular care. Be aware of the potential for delayed onset of toxicity. Continuing or increasing tachycardia, the development of ectopic beats and persisting vomiting are warning signs of worse to come. Measure the plasma theophylline concentration if there is any clinical doubt about the severity of intoxication; repeated analyses may be necessary in severe cases.

Preventing absorption
The stomach should be emptied if the patient presents within 4 hours of the overdose. Prompt administration of oral activated charcoal is vital and repeated doses must be given regardless of vomiting, if necessary by nasogastric tube and with administration of antiemetics. Whole-bowel irrigation (p. 42) appears to be an effective method of preventing absorption of sustained-release theophylline whereas volunteer studies suggest that catharsis induced by osmotic laxatives (without charcoal) may enhance absorption.

Supportive
Vomiting tends to be an intractable feature of theophylline intoxication of any severity and the usual antiemetics are frequently ineffective. The role of ondansetron in this situation has not been defined. Haematemesis may require blood transfusion but both cimetidine and ranitidine are contraindicated since they slow the metabolism of theophylline. Protection of the airway and maintenance of adequate ventilation are necessary if consciousness is impaired. Severe hypertension may respond to an intravenous beta-blocker or nifedipine.

Cardiotoxicity
The cardiac rhythm should be monitored continuously and dysrhythmias treated appropriately. In non-asthmatic patients, marked supraventricular tachycardia should be controlled with beta-adrenoceptor blockers. Large amounts may be required to produce adequate competition for receptor sites and the dose must be titrated against the clinical response. Ventricular dysrhythmias are treated similarly.

Control of convulsions
A combination of coma, convulsions and vomiting is particularly hazardous. In such situations it is advisable to paralyse, intubate and ventilate the patient rather than give parenteral anticonvulsants which may be required in large doses. If this approach is adopted, cerebral function should be monitored continuously and anticonvulsants given as necessary. Assisted ventilation also allows rapid correction of hyperventilation and respiratory alkalosis which contributes to the intracellular movement of potassium. For similar reasons it is important not to overcorrect any metabolic acidosis.

Correction of hypokalaemia
The increased potassium gradient across cell membranes may be important in the genesis of cardiac dysrhythmias and it seems reasonable to correct marked hypokalaemia (<2.8 mmol/l). This may be achieved by giving a non-selective beta-adrenoceptor blocker such as propranolol or by infusing potassium chloride. The latter approach carries the risk of hyperkalaemia during recovery from poisoning.

Elimination techniques
The plasma half-life of theophylline can be considerably shortened by repeated doses of oral activated charcoal which, provided they are tolerated, can be as effective as charcoal or resin haemoperfusion. If repeat-dose oral charcoal is not possible, charcoal haemoperfusion should be considered, particularly in grade 3 and 4 intoxication (as

defined above) and if plasma theophylline concentrations exceed 100 mg/l (770 µmol/l).

Prognosis

Severe poisoning with theophylline and its derivatives carries a significant mortality which is higher with acute overdosage than chronic intoxication. Most patients who die have grade 4 or, less commonly, grade 3 toxicity with plasma theophylline concentrations above 100 mg/l. Repeated convulsions and cardiac arrest indicate a poor prognosis.

References

Al-Shareef AH, Buss DC, Allen EM *et al*. The effects of charcoal and sorbitol (alone and in combination) on plasma theophylline concentrations. *Hum Exp Toxicol* 1990; **9**: 179–182.

Burkhart KK. Intravenous propranolol reverses hypertension after sympathomimetic overdose: two case reports. *Clin Toxicol* 1992; **30**: 109–114.

Janss GJ. Acute theophylline overdose treated with whole bowel irrigation. *SDJ Med* 1990; **43**: 7–8.

Jarvie DJ, Thompson AM, Dyson EH. Laboratory and clinical features of self-poisoning with salbutamol and terbutaline. *Clin Chim Acta* 1987; **168**: 313–322.

Sessler CN. Theophylline toxicity: clinical features of 116 cases. *Am J Med* 1990; **88**: 567–576.

Thyroxine and triiodothyronine

General considerations

Acute overdosage with thyroid hormones is seldom reported, probably because it rarely causes serious effects. Most episodes involve thyroxine (T_4) but there have been cases of acute overdosage with triiodothyronine (T_3).

Features

Only a minority of patients develop significant toxicity after acute overdosage with thyroid hormones. Symptoms develop within a few hours with T_3 but take 3–6 days following overdosage with T_4.

The principal effects are on the CNS and heart. Mental confusion, agitation, irritability and hyperactivity are common with mydriasis, tachycardia, tachypnoea and pyrexia. Other features of thyrotoxicosis, including atrial fibrillation, sweating, loose stools, lid retraction and prominence of the eyes appear to be uncommon. Convulsions developed in one child. In most cases toxic features abate in the same time as they take to develop.

The relatively benign and short-lived course of T_3 overdosage probably reflects its much shorter plasma half-life.

Thyroid function test abnormalities

Serum concentrations of hormones depend on the dose ingested and the time since ingestion and may be many times physiological values. Thyroid-stimulating hormone concentrations and I^{131} uptake are depressed within a few days but return to normal within 2 weeks. A normal serum T_4 more than 6 hours after ingestion precludes the possibility of delayed toxicity.

Management

The stomach should be emptied if more than 0.5 mg has been ingested by a child or more than 2 mg by an adult within 4 hours. Charcoal is indicated in children who have taken more than 3 mg. Blood should be taken 6–12 hours after ingestion for estimation of T_4 and T_3 concentrations. Patients with normal results may be discharged without follow-up. Those seen early and found to have high T_4 concentrations should be reviewed for evidence of toxicity on the fourth or fifth day postingestion.

Oral propranolol will rapidly control all the features of overdosage, the dose being titrated against the response in individual cases. Treatment should only be necessary for 5–6 days after the onset of toxic features.

Plasmapheresis has been used to enhance the elimination of T_4 after overdosage but is unnecessary and extravagant when morbidity is so low and beta-adrenoceptor blocking drugs so effective.

References

Berkner PD, Starkman H, Person N. Acute L-thyroxine overdose; therapy with sodium ipodate: evaluation of clinical and physiologic parameters. *J Emerg Med* 1991; **9**: 129–131.

Lin T-H, Kirkland RT, Kirkland JL. Clinical features and management of overdosage with thyroid drugs. *Med Toxicol* 1988; **3**: 264–272.

Mandel SH, Magnusson AR, Burton BT *et al.* Massive levothyroxine ingestion. *Clin Pediatr* 1989; **28**: 374–376.

Toiletries and cosmetics

General considerations

Toiletries and cosmetics are readily accessible in most homes and it is hardly surprising that they should be commonly involved in childhood 'poisoning'. Toilet articles frequently contain several different

Table 4.7 The usual principal constituents of common toilet preparations and cosmetics

Preparations	Constituents
*Skin preparations**	
Aftershave lotion	Ethanol
Colognes	Ethanol
Deodorants	Aluminium or zinc salts
Eye and face make-up	Numerous, non-toxic
Hand cream	Lanolin
Lipstick	Waxes, oils, dyes
Perfumes	Ethanol
Shaving cream	Salts of fatty acids
Hair preparations	
Hair lacquer	Ethanol
Hair remover	Potassium thioglycolate
Shampoo (liquid)	Lanolin, lauric diethanolamine, triethanolamine lauryl sulphate
Nail preparations	
Nail varnish	Toluene, ethanol, isopropanol, ethyl acetate
Nail varnish remover	Acetone, ethyl acetate, isopropanol
Bath preparations	
Bath crystals and cubes	Sodium carbonate and phosphate
Bubble bath solutions	Sodium lauryl ether sulphate

* Soaps are considered on p. 213.

potentially toxic compounds in relatively low concentrations. The usual principal constituents of the most common are listed in Table 4.7. Many are innocuous but others such as perfumes, colognes, aftershave lotions, mouth washes, hair removers, nail varnish and nail varnish removers are potentially toxic. The risk of consuming dangerous quantities is reduced by packaging them in relatively small volumes. However, this is not a protection with acetonitrile-containing solutions for removing artificial nails and bromates in neutralizers for permanent hair waves which have been a cause for recent concern.

Features

In general, ingestion of toiletries and cosmetics produces very few symptoms. Liquid shampoos, hand creams and lotions, lipstick, eye and face make-up, shaving cream and bubble bath soaps would have to be taken in fairly large amounts to cause problems. At worst there may be a little nausea and vomiting. Alimentary symptoms are more likely to follow consumption of thioglycolate-containing hair removers and bath salts.

Preparations containing ethanol (aftershave lotions, colognes, perfumes, mouth washes and hair lacquers) are amongst the most common toiletries ingested by children but serious intoxication (p. 119) is unlikely. Occasionally, however, they are taken as cheap forms of alcohol by alcoholics.

The toluene and acetone contained in nail varnish and nail varnish removers are also potential causes of serious poisoning with CNS depression, hepatic and renal necrosis and cardiac dysrhythmias in extreme cases (see pp. 223 and 61), although features of this severity rarely occur after accidental poisoning in childhood.

Acute pulmonary oedema has been described in children after inhalation of large quantities of talc-containing powders and a few deaths have resulted.

Products containing acetonitrile cause cyanide intoxication (p. 110) and bromates deafness and renal failure.

Management

Unless there is good evidence that a large quantity of a toilet or cosmetic preparation has been ingested there is little merit in trying to empty the stomach. Even symptomatic treatment is unlikely to be required. A short period of observation may be advisable to detect toxicity. In rare patients in whom consciousness is impaired or renal or hepatic damage has occurred treatment is supportive and conventional. Cyanide poisoning should be managed as on p. 111. Intravenous sodium thiosulphate converts bromate to bromide which can then removed by dialysis, the need for which should be judged from plasma bromide concentrations.

References

Geller RJ, Ekins BR, Iknoian RC. Cyanide toxicity from acetonitrile-containing false nail remover. *Am J Emerg Med* 1991; **9**: 268–270.

Hornfeldt CS. A report of ethanol poisoning in a child: mouthwash versus cologne, perfume and after-shave. *Clin Toxicol* 1992; **30**: 115–121.

Lichtenberg R, Zeller WP, Gatson R *et al.* Bromate poisoning. *J Pediatr* 1989; **114**: 891–894.

Losek JD, Rock AL, Boldt RR. Cyanide poisoning from a cosmetic nail remover. *Pediatrics* 1991; **88**: 337–340.

Pairaudeau PW, Wilson RG, Hall MA *et al.* Inhalation of baby powder: an unappreciated hazard. *Br Med J* 1991; **114**: 1200–1201.

Scherger DL, Wruk KM, Kulig KW *et al.* Ethyl alcohol containing cologne, perfume and after shave. Ingestions in children. *Am J Dis Child* 1988; **142**: 630–632.

Turchen SG, Manoguerra AS, Whitney C. Severe cyanide toxicity from the ingestion of an acetonitrile-containing cosmetic. *Am J Emerg Med* 1991; **9**: 264–267.

Vitamins

General considerations

Preparations containing one or a mixture of vitamins are commonly consumed in acute overdosage by children while some adults take large doses on a long-term basis, e.g. pyridoxine (vitamin B_6) for pre-menstrual tension. In general, chronic oral overdosage is more likely to cause toxicity than acute overdosage and water-soluble vitamins (B, C and folate) cause fewer problems than the fat-soluble ones (A in particular and also D). Some compound formulations also contain iron salts which are a greater hazard (see p. 133).

Features

The vast majority of children consuming an acute overdose of vitamins will have no features. Vitamin A has the greatest potential for acute toxicity, the required doses for an infant being about 350 000 iu and for an adult, 1.5 million iu. Since most vitamin A-containing preparations have no more than 4000–5000 iu per capsule or 5 ml, it is apparent that a very large number of dosage units would have to be consumed to cause toxicity.

Acute excess of nicotinamide might cause flushing and headache secondary to vasodilatation.

Acute overdosage with vitamin D is unlikely to cause toxicity whereas chronic ingestion of large amounts will cause hypercalcaemia and all its related consequences. Similarly, long-term pyridoxine may cause peripheral neuropathy and other neurological features.

Management

Acute overdosage with vitamins does not usually require treatment. In the unlikely event of toxic features developing, supportive care is all that can be offered.

Volatile substance abuse

Acetone
Butane
Carbon tetrachloride
Chloroform
Ether
Fluorinated hydrocarbons
n-Hexane
Lighter fluid (paraffin hydrocarbons)

Methyl-ethyl-ketone
Methylene chloride
Petrol
Tetrachloroethylene
Toluene
Trichloroethane
Trichloroethylene

General considerations

Volatile substance abuse is the current term applied to the deliberate inhalation of such substances for pleasurable effects and replaces former names such as solvent abuse, solvent sniffing and glue sniffing since it is now appreciated that gases and non-solvents may be misused in this way. It is most commonly found among young male teenagers and it is often a group activity. Many, but by no means all, have a background of emotional instability and come from broken or disturbed homes. Their academic performance is often poor and truancy is common. Much older abusers are far from uncommon.

Compounds such as those listed above are highly lipid-soluble and therefore have marked effects on nervous tissue. They are available, singly or in combination, in a wide variety of household products including shoe cleaners, polishes, adhesive cements, spot and nail polish removers, dry cleaning agents, cigarette lighter fuels, paint thinners, hair lacquers, fire extinguishers, typewriter erasing fluids and antifreeze preparations. The substance is usually applied to a piece of cloth and held near the nose or emptied into a plastic bag, the opening of which is then gathered together and held over the nose and mouth. Solvents may be inhaled in this manner intermittently for several hours. Elimination from the body is principally through the respiratory system but some solvents are metabolized, mainly in the liver.

Features

Solvents are inhaled for the CNS excitation ('buzz') they produce before depressing the brain. In the early stages they induce a sense of well-being and exhilaration which may include auditory and visual hallucinations. Dizziness and ataxia are common and there may be sneezing and coughing due to mild irritation of the respiratory mucosa. Behaviour may become abnormal and is dependent partly on the previous personality of the individual and partly on the reaction and activities of the group as a whole.

Increasing exposure causes progressive impairment of consciousness with mental confusion, loss of self-control, ataxia, dysarthria and nystagmus leading to coma and occasionally convulsions. Severe hypoxia may develop and, if combined with halogenated hydrocarbons which sensitize the heart to endogenous catecholamines, may cause fatal cardiac dysrhythmias. A severe metabolic acidosis may occur.

Sniffers are unlikely to come to medical attention while acutely intoxicated unless they are caught in the act, are creating a disturbance or develop some serious acute complication such as deep coma. However they may present later with other features which result from particularly heavy or repeated exposure. These include jaundice and renal damage (toluene, carbon tetrachloride and other halogenated hydrocarbons), acute and chronic encephalopathy (petrol with its tetraethyl lead content), cerebellar degeneration (toluene), or a predominantly motor, mixed polyneuropathy (hexane). The incidence of these complications cannot be determined with any certainty but is probably very low.

Abuse during pregnancy may lead to premature labour, perinatal deaths and growth retardation. Later growth and development may also be delayed.

Management

Stopping inhalation is all the 'treatment' most sniffers require for acute intoxication. As a result most have improved considerably by the time they reach hospital but some may require sedation if in a state of panic or if still excited or rowdy. Unconscious patients require supportive measures to ensure a clear airway and adequate ventilation and oxygenation. They should also have arterial blood gas analysis carried out and any metabolic acidosis corrected.

Hepatocellular and renal damage should be assessed biochemically and treated conventionally. Administration of N-acetylcysteine (in doses recommended for paracetamol overdosage) may be helpful if there has been heavy exposure to carbon tetrachloride.

Prognosis

The prognosis for uncomplicated acute intoxication is excellent and complete recovery can be expected within a few hours of stopping solvent exposure. Renal and hepatic damage is reversible but long-term neurological complications are unlikely to improve significantly. Abstinence from further solvent abuse is vitally important. Fortunately, neuropsychological impairment is unlikely in the great majority of children.

References

Ashton CH. Solvent abuse. Little progress after 20 years. *Br Med J* 1990; **300**: 135–136.

Chalmers EM. Volatile substance abuse. *Med J Aust* 1991; **154**: 269–274.

Cunningham SR, Dalzell GWN, McGirr P *et al*. Myocardial infarction and primary ventricular fibrillation after glue sniffing. *Br Med J* 1987; **294**: 739–740.

David NJ, Wolman R, Milne FJ *et al*. Acute renal failure due to trichloroethylene poisoning. *Br J Industr Med* 1989; **46**: 347–349.

Köppel C, Lanz H-J, Ibe K. Acute trichloroethylene poisoning with additional ingestion of ethanol – concentrations of trichloroethylene and its metabolites during hyperventilation therapy. *Intens Care Med* 1988; **14**: 74–76.

Roberts MJD, McIvor RA, Adgey AAJ *et al*. Asystole following butane gas inhalation. *Br J Hosp Med* 1990; **44**: 294.

Symposium. Volatile substance abuse. *Hum Toxicol* 1989; **8**: 255–334.

Taverner D, Harrison DJ, Bell GM. Acute renal failure due to interstitial nephritis induced by 'glue sniffing' with subsequent recovery. *Scot Med J* 1988; **33**: 246–247.

Wilkins-Haug L, Gabow PA. Toluene abuse during pregnancy: complications and perinatal outcomes. *Obstet Gynecol* 1991; **77**: 504–509.

Warfarin and superwarfarins

Superwarfarins

Brodifacoum	Coumatetralyl
Bromadiolone	Difenacoum
Chlorophacinone	Flocoumafen

General considerations

Warfarin is a widely used anticoagulant which competes with vitamin K, thereby blocking hepatic synthesis of factors II, VII, IX and X. Accidental and intentional acute poisoning are much less common than therapeutic overdosage. Occasionally, ingestion is not disclosed, causing diagnostic difficulty.

Warfarin is also the active ingredient of some rodenticides but is present in such small quantities that large amounts would have to be eaten by a human before serious poisoning developed. Resistance of rodents to warfarin has led to the introduction of 'superwarfarins' which act in the same manner but which are distinguished by their extremely long duration of action (weeks or months). Fortunately human poisoning with them is uncommon.

Features

Individual susceptibility to warfarin varies considerably and may be influenced by interaction with other drugs being taken concomitantly. Spontaneous bleeding is the only important consequence of acute warfarin poisoning and usually occurs from the nose, gums and gastrointestinal and urinary tracts. Less commonly there may be haemorrhage into the skin and brain. However, even in overdosage, warfarin takes 24–60 hours to exert its maximum anticoagulant effect and most patients will present, asymptomatic, long before haemorrhage is likely.

Plasma warfarin concentrations

Plasma warfarin concentrations of up to 30 mg/l have been reported after deliberate self-poisoning and decay with a half-life of 24–72 hours. The usual therapeutic range is 1–3 mg/l.

Management

The value of gastric emptying in acute warfarin overdosage is uncertain and unless a very large amount has been consumed it is probably better to rely on repeated administration of adsorbents such as cholestyramine which not only prevent absorption but also shorten the plasma half-life of drug already absorbed. Gastric emptying is probably advisable in addition to adsorbents after ingestion of superwarfarins because of their very prolonged duration of action.

Management thereafter depends on the amount ingested and whether or not the patient is on long-term anticoagulants, rapid reversal of which could be life-threatening (e.g. patients with prosthetic heart valves).

Patients not on long-term anticoagulants
If it is thought that only a small amount has been ingested, it is probably safe to take no further action but measure the prothrombin time at about 36–48 hours. Alternatively, vitamin K_1 could be given intravenously as a prophylactic measure. Unless given early, intramuscular injections are best avoided because of the risk of haematoma formation. Clearly, vitamin K_1 is indicated if significant, asymptomatic prothrombin time prolongation has occurred. If bleeding is already evident, fresh frozen plasma will be necessary for immediate control since vitamin K_1 will require about 24 hours to be effective. The need for repeated doses of vitamin K will depend on the compound involved and be decided according to prothrombin time measurements.

Patients on long-term anticoagulants
Intravenous infusion of fresh frozen plasma is also the treatment of choice when it is undesirable to completely reverse the anticoagulant effect of warfarin. If possible the prothrombin time should be kept at 2–3 times the control. It is essential to keep the patient under surveillance for several days because of the long plasma half-life of the drug. Warfarin should be restarted when fresh frozen plasma is no longer required and the prothrombin ratio is just slightly greater than the optimum for treatment.

References

Routh CR, Triplett DA, Murphy MJ *et al*. Superwarfarin ingestion and detection. *Am J Hematol* 1991; **36**: 50–54.

Smolinske SC, Scherger DL, Kearns PS *et al*. Superwarfarin poisoning in children: a prospective study. *Pediatrics* 1989; **84**: 490–494.

Wallace S, Paull P, Worsnop C *et al*. Covert self poisoning with brodifacoum, a 'superwarfarin'. *Aust NZ Med J* 1990; **20**: 713–715.

Weitzel JN, Sadowski JA, Furie BC *et al*. Surreptitious ingestion of a long-acting vitamin K antagonist/rodenticide, brodifacoum: clinical and metabolic studies of three cases. *Blood* 1990; **76**: 2555–2559.

Water hemlock and hemlock water dropwort

General considerations

Water hemlock and hemlock water dropwort are members of the highly poisonous *Cicuta* and *Oenanthe* genera of the Umbelliferae family of plants. Poisoning usually results from ingestion of the roots in mistake for parsnips and as little as one rhizome may be fatal for an adult. The subspecies involved in poisoning episodes in Europe and North America differ but contain either cicutoxin or oenanthotoxin which are unsaturated, 17-carbon, aliphatic alcohols.

Features

Symptoms commonly start within 1 hour of ingestion with malaise, nausea, hypersalivation, vomiting and abdominal cramps. The patient may be aware of palpitations but the most dramatic features of poisoning are extensor muscle spasms, opisthotonus and convulsions. The pupils are often dilated and cyanosis and pyrexia may be present. Both bradycardia and tachycardia have been described and although electrocardiogram changes may be found, they tend to be non-specific. Rare signs include parotid enlargement and flushing of the skin with subsequent desquamation.

There may be a polymorph leucocytosis and severe metabolic acidosis. High serum creatine phosphokinase and aspartate aminotransferase values occur commonly. Elevation of the former may be due to repeated convulsions but a toxic myositis has been postulated. Jaundice (in rare cases) and hypoprothrombinaemia suggest that hepatocellular damage may account for the raised aspartate aminotransferase.

Management

There is no specific treatment for water hemlock poisoning. The stomach should be emptied and convulsions controlled (p. 54). Other features should be treated symptomatically. Dantrolene may have a role if muscle tone is greatly increased. Otherwise, curarization and ventilation may be required.

Prognosis

Water hemlock poisoning carries a much higher mortality than most plant poisonings but if convulsions and extensor spasms can be controlled the patient is usually considerably improved within 12 hours. There may be fever and muscle pain and weakness for a few days after recovery. Long-term mental impairment with electroencephalogram changes has been reported.

References

Ball MJ, Flather ML, Forfar JC. Hemlock water dropwort poisoning. *Postgrad Med J* 1987; **63**: 363–365.
Landers D, Seppi K, Blauer W. Seizures and death on a white river float trip. *West J Med* 1985; **142**: 637–640.
O'Mahony S, Fitzgerald P, Whelton MJ. Poisoning by hemlock water dropwort. *Ir J Med Sci* 1987; **156**: 241.

Yew

General considerations

Various types of yew are commonly cultivated including *Taxus baccata* (the English yew), *T. canadensis* (the American yew) and *T. cuspidata* (the Japanese yew). The common name of the American yew, ground hemlock, is unfortunate since it is totally unrelated to the true hemlocks (*Conium* spp).

All parts of the yew are poisonous including the berries which comprise a single seed all but enclosed in an attractive fleshy red cup. The toxic principles, taxane alkaloids, have actions similar to cardiac glycosides and are well-absorbed, but the gastrointestinal features of poisoning may be due to irritant oils. Poisoning with yew berries is uncommon.

Features

Although poisoning with yew berries can be extremely serious and it has been claimed that death is sudden and survival unlikely, a French review reported symptoms in only 5 out of 33 alleged ingestions. The usual features of poisoning include vomiting and abdominal pain with diarrhoea. Convulsions and impairment of consciousness may occur with respiratory depression. The lethal effects, however, are those on the heart where depression of myocardial contractility and conductivity lead to complete heart block with broad-complex bradycardia and profound hypotension. Ventricular tachycardia and fibrillation may follow.

Management

The potential consequences of ingestion of parts of the yew tree are so serious that it would seem wise to empty the stomach if more than two or three berries have been ingested within 4 hours. Problems should then be dealt with as they arise. Cardiac pacing and inotropic support may be necessary if serious bradycardia develops and, failing that, digoxin-specific Fab fragment antibodies should be given as it has been suggested that they may cross-react with taxane alkaloids.

References

Cummins RO, Haulman J, Quan L *et al*. Near-fatal yew berry intoxication treated with external cardiac pacing and digoxin-specific FAB antibody fragments. *Ann Emerg Med* 1990; **19**: 38–43.

Yersin B, Frey J-G, Schaller M-D *et al*. Fatal cardiac arrhythmias and shock following yew leaves ingestion. *Ann Emerg Med* 1987; **16**: 1396–1397.

Zidovudine

General considerations

The increasing prevalence of acquired immune deficiency syndrome (AIDS) is likely to be associated with more people taking zidovudine and, consequently, overdoses of it.

Features

Information on overdosage with zidovudine is limited but toxicity appears to be relatively minor. Reported non-haematological effects include ataxia, nystagmus and convulsions. Minor increases of plasma transaminase activity have occurred but serious liver damage has not. Leucopenia and thrombocytopenia may develop but reduction of the red cell count appears to be more likely.

Management

Activated charcoal should be given, the patient's peripheral blood picture monitored and appropriate supportive measures instituted if indicated. Convulsions may require control with intravenous diazepam and a clear airway and adequate ventilation should be ensured.

Reference

Lafeuillade A, Poizot-Martin I, Dhiver C *et al*. Zidovudine overdose: a case with bone-marrow toxicity. *AIDS* 1991; **5**: 116–117.

Poisons information services

Eire

Dublin	Poisons Information Centre	0001–379966
	Beaumont Hospital	

England

Birmingham	West Midlands Poisons Unit	021–554 3801
	Dudley Road Hospital	
Leeds	Leeds Poisons Information Service	0532–430715
	General Infirmary	
London	National Poisons Information Service	071–635 9191
Newcastle	Northern Regional Drug &	091–232 5131
	Therapeutics Centre	

Northern Ireland

Belfast	Northern Ireland Drugs and Poisons	0232–240503
	Information Service	
	Royal Victoria Hospital	

Scotland

Edinburgh	Scottish Poisons Information Bureau	031–229 2477
	Royal Infirmary	

Wales

Cardiff	Welsh National Poisons Unit	0222–709901
	Llandough Hospital	

Appendix 2

Useful reference books

Ellenhorn MJ, Barceloux DG. *Medical Toxicology*. New York: Elsevier, 1988.

Gosselin RE, Smith RP, Hodge HC. *Clinical Toxicology of Commercial Products*, 5th edn. Baltimore: William & Wilkins, 1984.

Haddad LM, Winchester JF. *Poisoning and Drug Overdose*. Philadelphia: WB Saunders, 1990.

Hayes WJ, Laws ER. *Handbook of Pesticide Toxicology*. San Diego: Academic Press, 1991.

Martindale. The Extra Pharmacopoeia, 29th edn. London: The Pharmaceutical Press, 1989.

Proctor NH, Hughes JP, Fischman ML. *Chemical Hazards in the Workplace*, 2nd edn. Philadelphia: JB Lippincott, 1988.

Spoerke DG, Smolinske SC. *Toxicity of Houseplants*. Boca Raton: CRC Press, 1990.

The technique of gastric lavage

1 Before starting ensure that powerful suction apparatus is present and functioning. This may be required to remove gastric contents regurgitated around the stomach tube and should be capable of coping rapidly with large volumes.

2 Lie the patient in the left lateral position on a trolley.

3 Raise the foot of the trolley by 15–20 cm.

4 Lubricate and pass a stomach tube. Because of anxieties about the possible transmission of viral diseases by this procedure, the tube should preferably be of the disposable polyethylene variety and size 36 CH or 40 CH with an external diameter of approximately 14 mm should be used in adults. This size of tube is sufficiently large to be unlikely to pass through the vocal cords and is sufficiently firm (without being inflexible) to be passed without much cooperation from the patient.

5 Confirm that the end of the tube is in the stomach by aspirating or blowing some air down the tube while auscultating over the stomach. Use disposable plastic stomach tubes for drug addicts or others suspected of having had hepatitis.

6 Siphon off the gastric contents before carrying out lavage.

7 Perform gastric lavage by connecting the tube to a large funnel (using 1 m rubber or plastic hose) and by pouring 300 ml aliquots of tepid tap water down the stomach tube and then siphoning it off. Repeat the procedure until the returning fluid is clear of tablet particles. The efficiency of this technique may be improved by gently massaging over the left hypochondrium to aid the dislodgement and mixing of tablet fragments trapped in mucosal folds.

8 Once the effluent is clear withdraw the tube, taking care to occlude it completely between the fingers so that fluid left in the tube will not flood out when the end leaves the oesophagus and enters the pharynx. This simple measure should help reduce the danger of aspiration into the lungs. The suction apparatus may be needed.

Common names used by addicts

A	amphetamine
Acid	LSD
ADAM	methylenedioxyamphetamine
Amphet	amphetamine
Angel dust	phencyclidine
Aurora borealis	phencyclidine
Barbs	barbiturates
Beast	LSD
Bennies	amphetamine
Bernice	cocaine
Bhang	cannabis
Black tar	heroin
Blotter acid	LSD
Blow	cocaine
Blue caps	LSD
Blue drops	LSD
Blues	amphetamine
Boy	heroin
Brown caps	LSD
Brown sugar	heroin
Bush	cannabis
Busy bee	phencyclidine
C	cocaine
Cadillac	phencyclidine
Cadillac of drugs	cocaine
Champagne of drugs	cocaine
Charlie	cocaine
China white	fentanyl
Chinese	heroin
Chinese rock	heroin
CJs	phencyclidine
Coke	cocaine
Crap	heroin
Crystal	phencyclidine

Crystal joints	phencyclidine
Cube juice	morphine
Cycline	phencyclidine
Dama blanca	cocaine
Dana	heroin
Dexies	dexamphetamine
Dike	dipipanone
Doll	methadone
Dollies	methadone
Dolly	methadone
Dolophine	methadone
DOM	dimethoxymethylamphetamine
Dome dots	LSD
Domes	LSD
Dope	cannabis
Dose	cocaine
Dots	LSD
Downers	barbiturates
DP (Durban poison)	cannabis
Dreamer	morphine
Dujie	heroin
Dust	phencyclidine
Dynamite	cocaine
Ecstasy	methylenedioxymethylamphetamine
Elephant	heroin
Elephant tranquillizer	phencyclidine
Embalming fluid	phencyclidine
EVE	methylenedioxy-N-ethylamphetamine
Flake	cocaine
Fuel	phencyclidine
Ganja	cannabis
Ghost	LSD
Gold dust	cocaine
Good	phencyclidine
Grass	cannabis
Green caps	LSD
Green gold	cocaine
Green tea leaves	phencyclidine
H	heroin
Hagga	cannabis
Happy dust	cocaine
Happy sticks	cannabis/phencyclidine cigarettes
Happy trails	cocaine
Hard stuff	morphine

Harry	heroin
Hash	cannabis resin
Hash oil	cannabis oil
Hawk	LSD
Hit	cocaine
Hocus	morphine
Hog	phencyclidine
Horse	heroin
Horse tracks	phencyclidine
Ice	cocaine
Jam	cocaine
Joint	cannabis
Joy powder	heroin
Joy sticks	cannabis/phencyclidine cigarettes
Junk	heroin
Killer weed	phencyclidine
KJ	phencyclidine
Lady	cocaine
LBJ	phencyclidine
Leaf	cocaine
Line	cocaine
Liquid lady	cocaine/alcohol
Love pill	methylenedioxyamphetamine
M	morphine
Marijuana	cannabis
Mary Jane	cannabis
MDMA	methylenedioxymethylamphetamine
Mexican brown	heroin
Microdots	LSD
Miss Emma	morphine
Mist	phencyclidine
MJ	cannabis
Monkey	morphine
Monkey tranquillizer	phencyclidine
Morf	morphine
Morpho	morphine
Nembies	pentobarbitone
Noise	heroin
Orange wedges	LSD
Paki	cannabis
Paper acid	LSD
Paradise	cocaine
PCP	phencyclidine
Peace	phencyclidine

Peace pill	phencyclidine
Peace weed	phencyclidine
Persian	heroin
Pimp's drug	cocaine
Pink drops	LSD
Poor man's speedball	heroin/amphetamine
Pot	cannabis
Puff	cannabis
Purple haze	LSD
Purple wedges	LSD
Reefer	cannabis
Resin	cannabis resin
Rock	heroin or cocaine
Rocket fuel	phencyclidine
Rock'n'roll	heroin
Rufus	heroin
Scuffle	phencyclidine
Seccies	quinalbarbitone
Sherman	phencyclidine
Shit	cannabis
Smack	heroin
Smoke	cannabis
Snort	cocaine
Snorts	phencyclidine
Snow	cocaine
Sodies	sodium amylobarbitone
Soma	phencyclidine
Speed	amphetamine and other stimulants
Speedball	cocaine with heroin
Speed for lovers	methylenedioxyamphetamine
Split	cannabis
Star spangled powder	cocaine
STP	dimethoxymethylamphetamine
Stuff	heroin
Sulph	amphetamine
Sunshine	LSD
Supergrass	phencyclidine
Superjoint	phencyclidine
Super kool	phencyclidine
Superweed	phencyclidine
Surfer	phencyclidine
TAC	phencyclidine
Tea	cannabis
Thai sticks	cannabis

Thing	heroin
TIC	phencyclidine
TNT	heroin
Toot	cocaine
Uppers	amphetamine
Wake ups	amphetamine
Weed	cannabis
White elephant	heroin
White junk	heroin
White lightning	LSD
White powder	phencyclidine
White stuff	heroin
Window panes	LSD
Yellow caps	LSD
Yellow drops	LSD
Yuppie psychedelic	methylenedioxymethylamphetamine
Zoom	phencyclidine

Conversion factors for drug concentrations

To convert:

Drug	Molar units	to	Mass units	Multiply by
Amitriptyline (base)	µmol/l		µg/l	277.4
Barbiturates				
amylobarbitoneb	µmol/l		mg/l	0.226
butobarbitone	µmol/l		mg/l	0.216
cyclobarbitone	µmol/l		mg/l	0.236
pentobarbitone	µmol/l		mg/l	0.226
phenobarbitone	µmol/l		mg/l	0.232
quinalbarbitoneh	µmol/l		mg/l	0.238
Carbamazepine	µmol/l		mg/l	0.236
Chlormethiazole (base)	µmol/l		mg/l	0.1615
Digoxin	nmol/l		µg/l	0.781
Ethanol	mmol/l		mg/l	46.0
Ethylene glycol				
Imipramine (base)	µmol/l		µg/l	230.4
Iron	µmol/l		µg/l	55.85
Isopropanol	mmol/l		mg/l	60.1
Meprobamate	mmol/l		mg/l	218.3
Methanol	mmol/l		mg/l	32.0
Paracetamol	mmol/l		mg/l	151.2
Phenytoin	µmol/l		mg/l	0.252
Quinine	µmol/l		mg/l	0.325
Salicylate	mmol/l		mg/l	138.1
Theophylline	µmol/l		mg/l	0.13

Molar values can be obtained by dividing mass values by the same factors.

Index

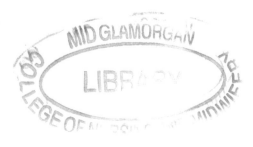